Women
& Beauty

Women & Beauty

By

SOPHIA LOREN

William Morrow and Company, Inc

Library of Congress Catalog Card Number: 84-60578

ISBN: 0-688-01394-5

Printed in Italy by Arnoldo Mondadori Editore, Verona

First U.S. Edition

1 2 3 4 5 6 7 8 9 10

Many thanks to Kathy Matthews whose close collaboration
and friendship made this book possible.

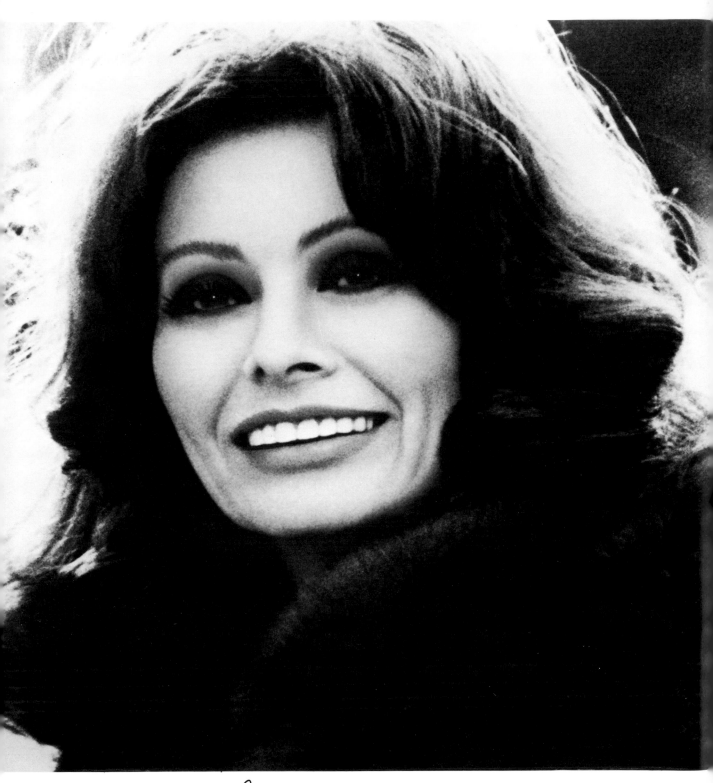

CONTENTS

INTRODUCTION

I have given the idea of beauty a great deal of thought for this book. The first thing I realized is that there is no one particular way for you to become beautiful, no matter what you may read elsewhere; unfortunately it is more complicated than that. But I have worked in a business that prizes beauty very highly. Being "professionally" beautiful has taught me a lot and I think that my experience can help you. My hope is that I will inspire you to think about beauty in a new way, help you to discover your own individual beauty, and teach you some beauty techniques that you can adapt to your own life.

I have tried here to speak only of those things I know. I can't pretend to tell what color a blonde should use on her eyes or what blouse will look well on a flat-chested woman. Instead, I hope to share with you what I have learned about beauty through my work, my experience and my travels. I have tried to talk about subjects that will be of use to all women. This is not a book of techniques, although I have included tips and suggestions whenever I can. My goal is to help you take a second, mature look at how a woman is beautiful.

The most exciting part of this mature approach to beauty is that it does not depend on possessing the dewy cheeks of a teenager or making up to disguise an imperfect nose. It depends on qualities available to us all: charm, warmth, wisdom and the intelligence and imagination you can bring to improving the way you look.

Some Thoughts on Beauty

A SECOND LOOK AT BEAUTY

When we think about beauty, we usually dwell on the mechanics – skin creams, hairdos, how to apply mascara. This is an important approach because, after all, most of us are always ready to learn some new trick that will make us more attractive. And these techniques do work. Nonetheless, what I propose to do in this book is to give a different approach to beauty, one that will serve women of all ages and of different natural gifts. My approach to beauty begins not with the face or figure but with the mind. If you can learn to use your mind as well as you use a powderpuff, you will become more truly beautiful.

As teenagers most of us are enthralled with makeup and hairstyles. This is a new world to us and a badge of our femininity and we spend hours at the mirror experimenting. But as time goes by, we limit our beauty explorations to a new color of lipstick or a new hairstyle. We become set in our ways. Our ideas about beauty have become formed and we move on to other pursuits. When we are shopping for a new dress or at the hairdresser, we might give some thought to the way we look, but we do so in a sporadic and disorganized way. This means that as adults we are left with ideas about beauty that haven't really changed since we were adolescents. As mature women, we still think that beauty is technique and too few of us progress beyond that notion.

I suggest that once the fervent explorations of our youth are past, it is time to take a new look at beauty. For mature beauty is very different from youthful beauty. It demands a different approach. Where youthful beauty is unconscious, mature beauty is knowing and sophisticated. It admits to effort. It is also richer and more complex.

Beauty is valuable. There is no doubt of that. We live in a world that prizes beauty and rewards those who are believed to be beautiful. This can seem most unfair until you come to understand what beauty really is and what part it plays in your life.

A journalist once said of me that my mouth is too large, my nose is too long, my chin and lips are too broad and yet the sum of the parts is somehow beautiful. I tell you this not to praise myself but simply to demonstrate that beauty doesn't exist as an ideal. There is a great deal you

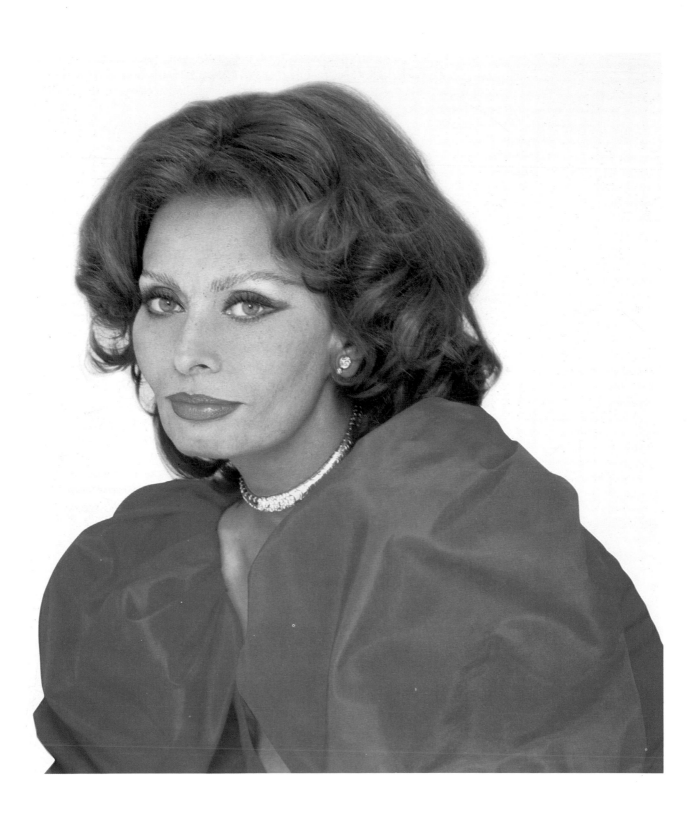

can learn about beauty that has nothing to do with cosmetics or hairdos or diet or exercise. If I can convince you of this, the techniques of beauty, important as they are, will fall into their proper place as enhancements, not essentials.

If you were to ask a half dozen people what they think makes a woman beautiful, you would probably get a list of specific features: a big smile, long, glossy hair, a firm, slim figure, perfect, glowing skin and so on. All these attributes are certainly beautiful and any woman would be glad to have them. Yet I believe that beauty is something more than this.

Perhaps you have heard it said that "beauty is only skin deep," or some such proverb, and you may not believe it. It sounds like a stuffy moral judgment or the sort of comfort a mother gives her plain daughter. But from my experience in a business obsessed with beauty I can tell you that this notion of beauty being something more than a list of features is true.

I am sure you can see it in your own life. Consider for a minute the women you know and see frequently and one or two will probably come to mind as being especially beautiful. But if you think about it, they are probably more attractive than beautiful. Because if you stop and examine these "beautiful" women you will almost surely see that something more than hair, eyes, skin and figure made them spring to mind. In fact, they may have some defects like a big nose or small eyes or a less-than-perfect complexion. Yet somehow they have convinced you, and probably most of the people in their lives, that they are beautiful.

You have to remember that the beauty business today is large and lucrative. It is a business that is forced to assume that ideal beauty is a reality, otherwise it couldn't possibly come to grips with the many different ways in which women are beautiful. To handle such diversity would be an overwhelming task and would rob the fashion world of the "freshness" of each season that adopts and promotes a new "ideal" beauty. It is easier – and more profitable – to tell people that all lips should be pale this year than to tell them that pale lipstick is being sold but not to buy it unless it is right for them and their old lipstick is worn out. It is largely for business reasons that fashions change so much from year to year, and the woman who is deemed "beautiful" this year is outdated the next.

But ideal beauty is a mirage. Altering your hairstyle to the "perfect" style for your face or discovering an extraordinary new night cream or eye shadow or this season's popular new dress designer will certainly alter your appearance, but real beauty is not just a matter of looking up-to-date. There is an element of beauty that has nothing to do with what you will see in most books and magazines. Once you have accepted this, you are ready to understand what makes a woman beautiful and to learn how you can cultivate your own beauty in the most effective way.

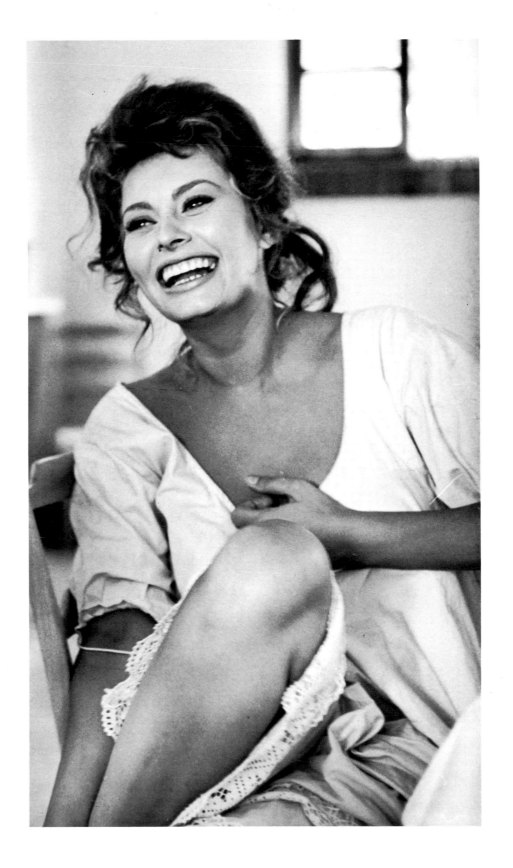

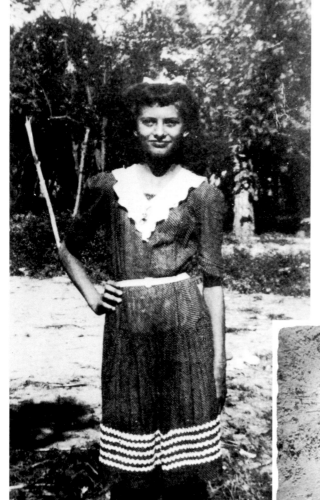

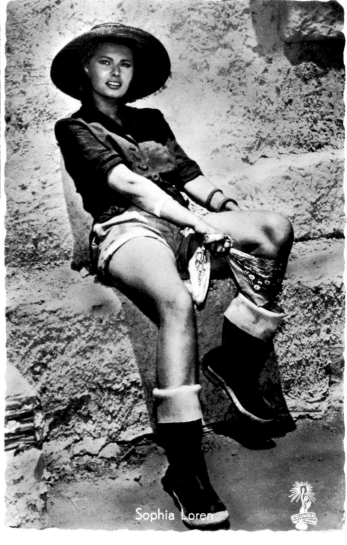

I wasn't always considered beautiful. When I was thirteen (above) my nickname was "Toothpick," when I began my career they called me "Giraffe."

Sophia Loren

In my opinion, there are two things you must recognize about beauty in order to achieve it: first, that it is within your reach, and second, that it is worth working for.

I think it is helpful to take a close look at the word "vanity" in order to convince yourself that beauty is within your reach.

Vanity and Beauty

I read not long ago that to be vain is to have too high an opinion of one's looks. This seemed correct to me and of no particular interest. But later the definition came back to mind, and the more I thought about it the more it seemed to me that it contained an important error. We know that vanity is foolish and therefore, according to this definition, if we are to avoid vanity we must have an accurate opinion of our appearance. But do we take the world's opinion of how we look and assume it is the truth? Do we count on others to let us know where we fit on the scale of perfection? I believe that this would be a great mistake.

You must be realistic about many things in life. If you are a bad driver, you shouldn't borrow someone's new Rolls-Royce. If you can't sing, you shouldn't inflict your arias on others. But no matter what others think, you must be convinced that, in your way, you are beautiful. What this amounts to is that in order to be beautiful, a woman must be vain. At first, the idea seems repulsive. Who, after all, would wish to be considered unrealistically pleased with her own looks? But give the idea a little more attention and I think you will understand what I mean and will come to agree with me.

As I said before, a collection of perfect features does not make for beauty. Perfect features, perfectly assembled, call to mind the cold proportions of a Greek statue, not a warm, desirable, beautiful woman. So if it is not conforming to an ideal of what is beautiful that makes a woman attractive, what is it? And what does this have to do with vanity?

Again, if you turn to your friends or even to women who appear in the media, you will see that the beautiful ones, those who catch your eye and make you delight in them and perhaps envy them, are the ones who believe that they are beautiful. Somehow they have discovered that they are beautiful, and they radiate the pleasure of their discovery, even though their features or their figures or their makeup are not perfect. You recognize immediately their confidence in their own appearance. Indeed, I am convinced that nothing makes a woman more beautiful than the belief that she is so.

When I began my career, my nickname was "Giraffe" because I was so tall and awkward. No one thought I was especially beautiful, but everyone knew right away that I was proud. In the beginning people were impressed with my confidence, and gradually they came to see it as beauty. On the other hand, I know a woman who is convinced that she is too tall; she is so self-conscious about her height that most of the time she looks as if she would like to disappear. All she thinks about is her height and that is all you notice about her. Unless her attitude changes, the sad fact is that although she is very pretty, she has no chance of being thought attractive.

And so we return to the idea of vanity. If to be vain is to have too high an opinion of your looks, then you all should learn to be vain – not in the vulgar, competitive sense, but with the healthy, positive conviction that you are beautiful. You must all, somewhere deep in your hearts, believe that you have a special beauty that is like no other and that is so valuable that you must not abandon it. Indeed, you must learn to cherish it. Later I will talk about some of the qualities that you need to think about if you are to have a healthy vanity, such as charm, self-confidence and style. But first I want to convince you of the importance of vanity for your own sense of beauty.

Though I, like everyone else, have made mistakes in discovering my own beauty, I can tell you of an instance early in my career when the vanity of a young girl served me well. When I first had the opportunity for a screen test, I was just a girl from nowhere eager for a chance to begin a career. After every screen test it was always the same story from the technicians: there is no way to make this girl look good – her nose is too long and her hips too broad. And would I think about trimming off just a bit of my nose?

In retrospect, I am surprised and proud of the vanity of the girl I was then. Though poor and anxious to begin work, I refused to alter anything. They would take me as I looked or not at all. I was very lucky that I didn't ruin my career at that moment. Eventually I profited by looking only like myself and not like what was fashionable years ago with certain film technicians in Rome. Though I made that decision instinctively, I realize now that a woman who believes with great conviction in her attractiveness will ultimately convince others that she is correct. And like my tall friend, a woman convinced of her ugliness will also convince others of it.

It is a lack of vanity that leads women in so many wrong directions in their quest for beauty. If you have a low opinion of your appearance, you are at the mercy of every salesperson and every hairdresser who wants to give you bad, if "fashionable," advice about how you should look. We have all seen women changing their look from season to season, trying to discover their beauty but always vulnerable to the world's opinion of their appearance. They, and we, need vanity in order to discover our genuine beauty.

Working Toward Beauty

Perhaps you are saying, "It is all very well, Sophia, for you to say that I must be vain and then, believing I am beautiful, I will be so. But it's not that easy for me." Of course, you are right if you hesitate at this point and tell yourself that beauty is more than belief. Yes, there is a mundane side to this, which brings me to my second point about beauty: that it is worth working for.

At first, this seems obvious – what woman would deny it? And yet . . . and yet . . . there seems to be a side to most women that refuses to recognize that it is worth the time and effort it takes to be beautiful. As I have said already, only the very young girl is effortlessly beautiful. She has a freshness and potential that are uniquely appealing. But don't envy her. It is immature to think that you can be beautiful forever without trying, that a freshly washed face and the most handy clothes will carry you through a lifetime.

I am afraid that the media help promote the idea of effortless beauty. We watch a film in which a woman wakes up in the early morning, her hair tousled but somehow perfect, her face dewy and radiant, her lashes dark seemingly without mascara, her lips naturally rosy. We are supposed to believe that a woman really looks this way in the first minutes of her day.

I know I don't look like that and you probably don't either. But we are made to feel that there is something wrong if we have to put effort into achieving our best look. Many women, understandably enough, rebel against this. They tell themselves that they won't bow to fashion and the dictates of beauty, that it is all impossible and frivolous and not worth the effort. They give up. They wear any old thing and see lipstick as a political weapon. Though I can understand this reaction, I think they are making a mistake. With a positive attitude, beauty is within the reach of every woman.

Don't be ashamed to take the necessary time to maintain your appearance: it is important to your own feelings of self-esteem and therefore will affect how the world reacts to you. I don't mean that spending hours on makeup and shopping and hairstyling is essential to beauty. I know many women who have brief and simple beauty routines that serve them very well. In this book you will learn about my beauty routines, and they are certainly not complicated or time-consuming. But no one arrives at such routines without effort.

I hope that I have convinced you to take your beauty seriously. I hope that you will, perhaps with the help of this book, discover what is beautiful about yourself. And then I hope that you will commit yourself to the effort that real beauty requires.

And finally, before I become too serious and ponderous, let me remind you that the pursuit of beauty is one of the great joys of being a woman. It should give you pleasure and it should be fun. When you try on a hat or an eyeliner, you see yourself in a new light. Knowing yourself a little better gives you confidence and even power. Working toward beauty should bring both joy and fulfillment.

Self-confidence

In 1959, I was making a film called *Heller in Pink Tights*. George Cukor was directing, and I was eager to work with him because he had a reputation as a "woman's director." Everyone said he had a special instinct about developing a woman's potential and had an eye for beauty. I expected him to spend a lot of time fussing with makeup and costume, and he certainly was demanding about these things. But gradually I came to learn that for him the soul of beauty was elsewhere. One day, in the course of explaining how a character should emphasize her attractiveness, he said something that I have never forgotten: "Beauty without self-confidence is less attractive than ugliness with self-confidence. If you are confident, you are beautiful."

Since then, time and time again I have seen Cukor's words demonstrated at parties, on film sets, or on the street: a woman without self-confidence will never be beautiful in a way that attracts others. I can't tell you exactly why this is so, but it is. Perhaps because we are all to some degree doubtful about ourselves, we look to others for certainty. This is as true for a woman who wants to be beautiful as it is for a politician who wants to lead men. If a woman seems convinced of her allure, we believe her and we are drawn to her.

Confidence is difficult to define, but we all know it when we see it. Sometimes it can be a woman who walks proudly down the street and attracts our eye even though she is not particularly pretty. Sometimes it is a man who, though very famous or important, is genuinely kind to those around him. In my opinion, self-confidence implies a balance between courage and self-control. True confidence is always marked by simplicity and sincerity. Confidence grows when you try to be yourself at your best.

You can build self-confidence by knowing yourself. That is not just a matter of counting your strengths. You must know your weaknesses as well. Self-confidence doesn't grow from perfection; that is out of the question. If you know your weaknesses, you can control them, not vice versa.

Confidence begins with experience. You act in a certain way and you meet with success, and the next time you are confident about how to act. I have found this to be true in so many cases. When faced with my first interview or my first television talk-show appearance, I was far from confident. But I tried to act as if I were completely calm and in control, and that helped me. The next time, I was truly confident even though I was still nervous; I had been through it before and I knew what to do.

As far as beauty is concerned, in order to be confident we must accept that the way we look and feel is our own responsibility. It can be hard to accept this today in a world which encourages us to put the blame for all our problems elsewhere – on our parents, friends, jobs. But unless you decide to

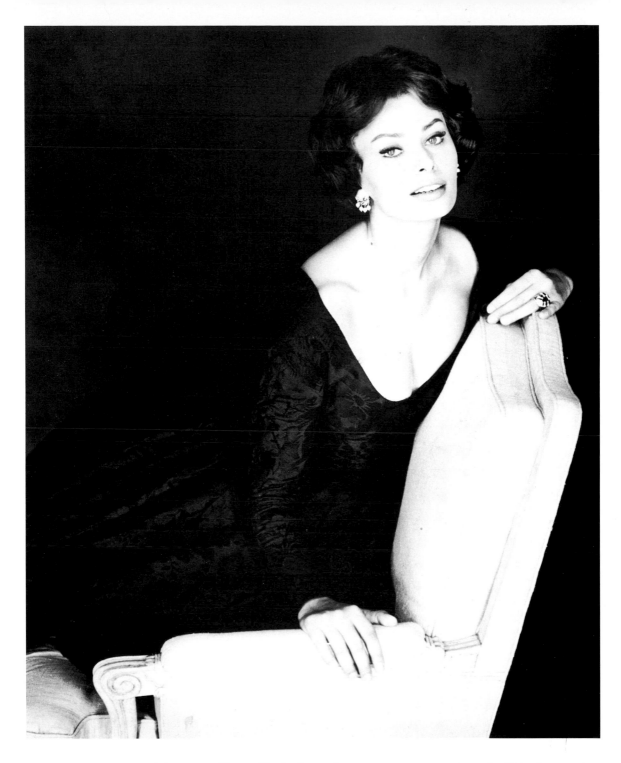

take a positive attitude toward your appearance, there is little hope of success. You can never be confident because you don't believe the matter is in your hands. Once you are convinced you have reason to be confident, the potential to be truly beautiful is yours.

The Pursuit

of

Beauty

DISCIPLINE AND BEAUTY

*D*iscipline is the key to success in so many areas of life. If you have no discipline, you will find it very hard to be beautiful. I am reminded of this constantly by the women I have met in my career who are considered beautiful. You may think that film stars or celebrities look the way they do without effort, but don't delude yourself. It is easy to think that if only you could have the most expensive products and technicians you would be beautiful too. Believe me, in almost every instance, the actress you see on the screen or the beautiful woman you pass on the street doesn't rely on experts to create her. They may improve her but they can't invent what is not there. The difference between the beautiful woman and the average woman is discipline.

There are two comforting factors in this harsh rule. First, discipline is the great equalizer. If a young woman is beautiful but has no discipline, she will lose her looks as she grows older. If a plain woman is disciplined she will undoubtedly become more beautiful with time.

The second comfort is that the more you develop discipline, the easier it becomes. I often find myself at lunches or dinners where there is an enormous amount of excellent food. It used to be difficult for me to say no to something, but now I am so accustomed to paying attention to whether or not I am really hungry that refusing a dessert or an extra helping is not an ordeal, it is just a fact of how I live my life. The same goes for exercise and shopping for clothes and so many other activities.

I know you won't believe me if I claim that it is always easy. It is a constant struggle to force yourself to do something you don't feel like doing. Sometimes, with exercise for example, I avoid action until I am almost sick with guilt. Then at the last moment before I sink into despair, I give myself a sort of mental slap and say, "OK, girl, you'd better get going right now or all is lost!" Then, once I have begun, it's all right, and the satisfaction that eventually comes is worth the agony beforehand.

I am reminded of a couple I saw one Sunday morning in Bürgenstock in Switzerland, where I live. They were walking arm in arm, perhaps on their way to church. They moved slowly; the man was stooped with age. But they were dressed in what must have been their best clothes, so neat and pressed, and he had a flower in his jacket lapel. I thought to myself, "That is a lifetime of discipline." To me they were enviable because the care they took with the details of their lives obviously gave them great pleasure.

Daily attention to beauty routines is one side of discipline. Another side is attention to recent developments in nutrition, hair care, makeup and fashion. This is less important than daily routines, but it has a beneficial effect. Even when, for example, you pick up a magazine in a doctor's office and read about a new kind of mascara or a good recipe and decide to try them, this is to the good. You don't have to be a scientist about the latest beauty developments, but having an open mind and a healthy curiosity will keep you up-to-date.

I enjoy looking at books and magazines and trying new ideas and products. This is a kind of play for me because I don't change my standard routines quickly, but I like to experiment and try something new now and again. Every once in a while I find a new technique or idea that I like and I adopt it permanently. But I think the main benefit of keeping an eye on new beauty ideas is that they are inspirational. When you are feeling low or unattractive or bored, looking at a book or magazine that exhorts you to improve yourself is very useful.

I am going to give you some suggestions on hair and makeup and other beauty routines. All of them demand discipline. Naturally no one can force you to change your ways and you shouldn't adopt my ideas if they are not right for you. But I want to say one thing before I begin. An excuse you should never use for neglecting yourself is lack of time. Sometimes we tell ourselves that we are too busy to do this or that, but really it is just an empty excuse. The only time that a woman may truly be too busy to look after herself is when she has a new baby at home. Otherwise you can always find time. I know it's hard. When you have family and work and other obligations, your time is not your own. But it isn't any easier for me to do these things than for you. Still, I get up an hour earlier, push myself away from the table, discipline myself to focus on the goal and not on the difficulty. Be very clear-headed about what you want from life and how you want to spend your time so that you don't allow an empty excuse to disguise lack of will.

Now, you have no excuse not to be beautiful, and you have my warm encouragement to proceed.

HAIR – THE VITAL ACCESSORY

*I*n the film *Madame Sans-Gêne*, which I made in 1960, I started out as a simple French washerwoman and ended as a duchess. My washerwoman hair was wild and disheveled; this made it easier for me to act with the passion and gusto that the role demanded. It was a hairdo that encouraged big gestures and a wild sweep of skirts in the dust. When I became a duchess, my hair was polished, styled. Likewise my gestures and expressions became more civilized and restrained. My every movement was controlled, like my hair.

Your hair can do the same for you – it can be a beauty accessory that helps you play whatever role your life demands with greater effectiveness and ease. I have always been impressed as an actress by how the accessories of a part – the costume, makeup and hairdo – can help to create the essence of a character. Even though you may not be an actress, you should be aware of how your most important natural accessory can affect not only your look but your spirit and even, to some degree, your approach to life.

A lot of attention is always given to the practical aspects of hair care. But I really think the most important asset about your hair is using it to express yourself and to fulfill an image of what you want to be. Some women will always want long hair because the way it falls against their necks makes them feel romantic; for others, the gamin look better suits their image.

When my sister Maria was young, I could always tell when she had fallen in love with another man because she would dye her hair a different color. Like most girls, she found that each man brought out something different in her and also in her hair. It became quite a joke between us. Whatever your personality and your fantasy, when you think about hair, first learn all the facts and then let your dreams and imagination come into play. After all, your hair is one of the most versatile accessories you have: you can change its color, its length and its style quite easily. And it is the only accessory you wear all the time.

Choosing the Right Hairstyle

A good hairstyle is usually the result of trial and error, and often the errors

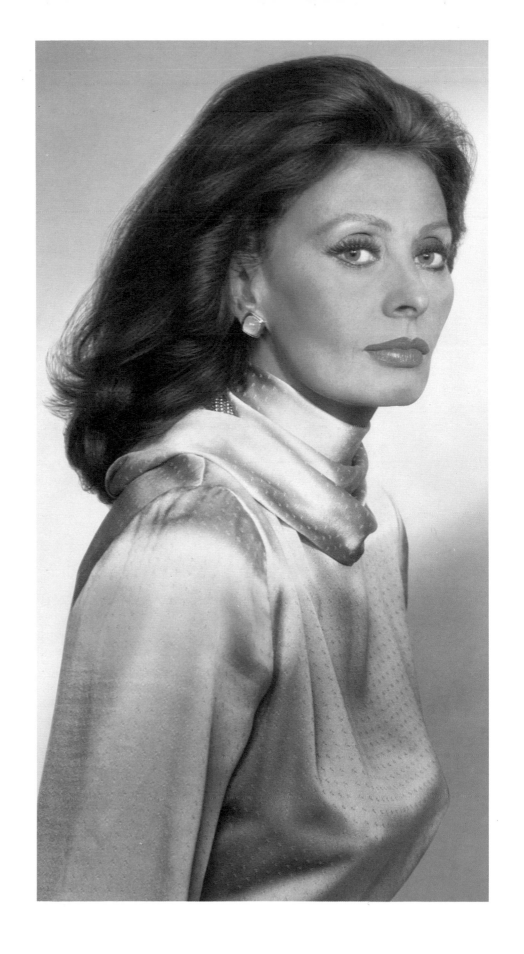

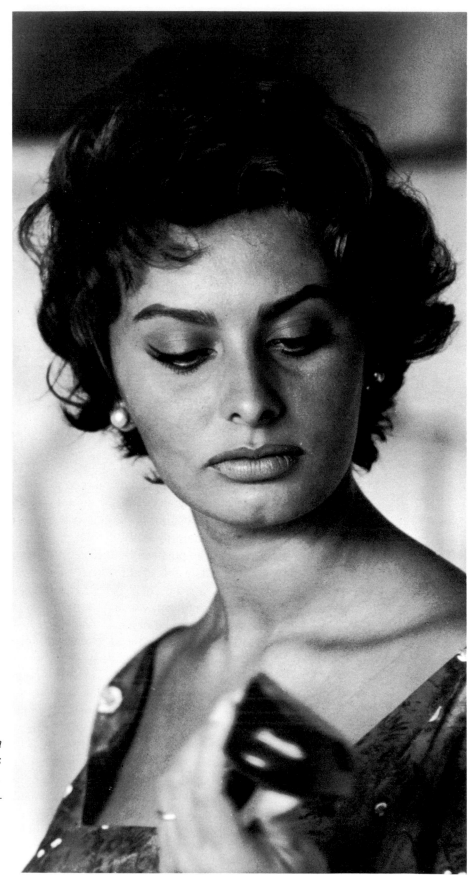

In the course of my film career I have had many different hairstyles, and I found that each one highlighted various aspects of my looks and my personality.

are painful because it takes months to correct them. We women are compelled to take all these risks with our hair for a very good reason: the right hairstyle can make a plain woman beautiful and a beautiful woman unforgettable. It is like a sweepstake, and every time you opt for a completely new style you are taking a chance on hitting the jackpot. Given the exciting possibilities and the potential anxiety, I think it makes sense to learn some facts and try to look at your own situation with some objectivity before making your next leap of faith at the hairdresser.

First of all, I believe that many of the "rules" of hairstyling are limiting. For example, you may hear that if you have a round face you should never wear bangs; or perhaps if you have fine hair you should never wear it long. But I have seen many women with very fine hair wearing it long, and they look wonderful. Likewise many "experts" may say that once a woman is in her thirties she should cut her hair, as long hair pulls the face down and makes it look older. This is another old-fashioned idea; some older women have beautiful long hair that should never be cut. Today there is room for every kind of look; however, some hairstyling advice hasn't caught up with the times.

Likewise, the rules for disguising features that are not perfect can be inhibiting. Very often some unusual feature that you have should be emphasized rather than hidden. I have read that if you have strong features, a more complicated hairdo is to your advantage because it puts your face into proportion. But I have strong features and I find I look much better with a simple hairdo. When I have been forced to wear complicated hairdos for film roles, everyone agrees that they do not flatter me.

One of the most important aspects of any hairstyle is comfort. I like a hairdo that I am barely aware of as I move through my day. It is distracting constantly to have to push your hair back or fix your bangs or smooth your crown. You should be able to comb your hair now and again and then forget about it. There is also a psychological aspect to a comfortable hairdo. If you have a look that suits you, you feel at ease. We can probably all think of times when we have had a hairstyle that was a mistake. It seems that such styles always look awkward; they are either too curly or too flat, or there is some other flaw. At the mercy of such a style you are always planning your day, and ultimately your life, so that you can do things when your hair looks good. A rainy day makes your heart sink because you know as soon as your smooth hairdo is exposed to humidity you'll look like a poodle. This is really no way to live. You should have a style that makes you feel at ease no matter what the weather, the time of day or the wind velocity.

Fashion is yet another force that can mislead us in choosing a hairstyle. It is fun to watch how styles change over the years. Every season a new look is promoted as "the" style every fashionable woman must have. One season the look is a short, boyish cut, and a few months later long, romantic curls are all the rage. What, I always wonder, happens to those girls with the short haircuts? Do they go into hiding while they wait for their hair to grow out?

I often look in magazines and see fashionable styles that I long to try, hairdos that are completely different from my usual smooth, simple look. Every now and again I will try one of them, but I always return to my regular style, which I think is both comfortable and flattering. People are always trying to get me to change my hairstyle by saying, "Oh, Sophia, you've had that style for so long. Why not try a short, curly look or a new color or something different?" I know their intentions are good, but now I always refuse. I believe that change just for the sake of change is pointless. If you ever see Greta Garbo today, you will notice that she looks beautiful – older, of course, but still beautiful. And she is wearing her hair just as she did forty years ago. Can you think of any reason for her to change? If you are happy with the style you have, stick with it. Experiment now and again, but if the experiment doesn't work, go back to the original.

Hair for Your Look and Your Life

When you choose a hairdo, there are two things you must take into consideration: your own personal look and your life-style. One woman who seems to have found the perfect hairstyle for her life and her look is Liza Minnelli. She has a unique, short, elfin cut that is her signature. It looks so pretty and right that you can't imagine her wearing any other hairstyle. And for a woman who performs with such energy and is so active, it must be very easy to take care of.

As far as your own look is concerned, the goal is to find a style that capitalizes on your own hair type while it flatters your face. The right hairstyle can do so much to improve your overall appearance that it is worth taking the time to find one. And you will only find it by experimenting.

Take into serious consideration your hair type when you are selecting a new cut. If you have very curly hair, work with it: don't pick a style that requires you to straighten your hair for it to look right. I remember in the late sixties, when everyone wanted to have long, straight hair, women with curly hair had theirs straightened regularly. In my opinion, nature knows what it is doing when it matches your face with your hair. Today when I see those women who used to straighten their hair with natural curls surrounding their faces, I really think they look much prettier. The curls flatter them in a way that straight hair never did. If your hair is as straight as fettuccine, it is easier to make a dramatic change because you can get a perm, but remember that a perm alters the basic structure of your hair. As with the women who straightened their hair in the sixties, you may find that if you perm your

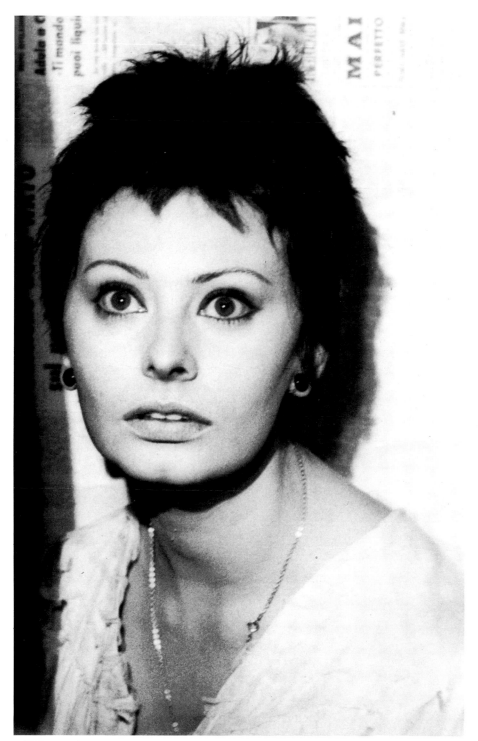

This gamin style suited my role as the young girl in Marriage, Italian Style. *By the end of the film I was a woman of fifty-five with a very different hairstyle.*

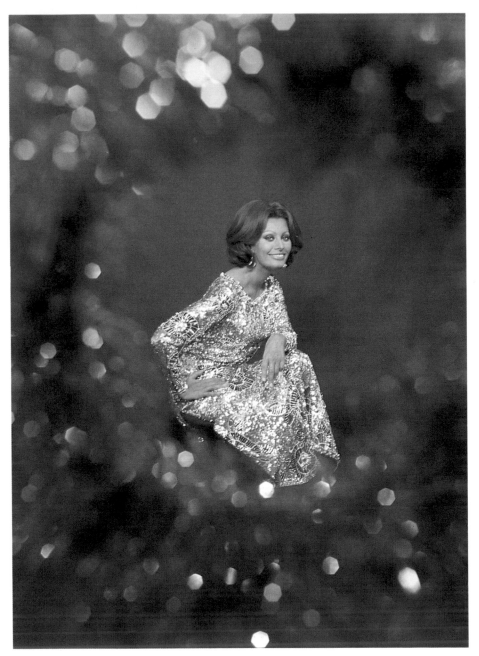

I always prefer a simple hairstyle, however formal the occasion.

naturally straight hair into a cloud of frizz, it may not work for your face.

Consider your figure and your stature when you judge a hairstyle. A full-length mirror is a must. If you are very short, you don't want to be overpowered by a big, fussy style. If you are tall or heavy, a very compact hairdo can make your head look too small and out of proportion. Just keep in mind that a hairstyle does not affect only your face but your whole body.

Earlier I mentioned life-style as a factor in choosing a haircut. Here is what I meant. If you are a mother with young children, your day is probably quite hectic. It would be foolish to choose a style that demands a great deal of attention. If you are a businesswoman, you need to project a certain neat, in-control look and a simple, straightforward style can help you achieve this. When you think about your life-style, don't forget the climate you live in. If you live in an area that constantly is either humid or quite dry, this might make a difference in the cut that will work for your type of hair.

Sometimes women who go out a great deal in the evening wonder if they should have a more elaborate hairstyle to go with their formal clothes. I think this idea is really outdated, and I advise you simply to find your own best look for daytime and, when the occasion demands, dress up the style with jewelry, hair ornaments or ribbons. Some of the prettiest evening styles are very simple, with a flower or perhaps a single piece of costume jewelry to add interest.

Finally, practical Sophia reminds you to consider cost. Some hairstyles, particularly short cuts, demand that you visit your hairdresser quite frequently. Over a period of time this can become expensive, and you could look a bit ragged at the edges as you try to save some money by skipping the hairdresser. Be realistic about what you can afford. A good hair stylist should be able to tell you in advance how often you'll need to visit the salon, and you should be a little hard-headed and figure out how much the hairdo is going to cost.

How Not to Choose a New Hairstyle

Choosing a hairstyle can be an emotional event in any woman's life. It is hard to be calm and collected when you are on the verge of looking much better or, heaven forbid, much worse than you already look. This inevitable tension concerning a new hairstyle is one thing. But some of us make the mistake of using an emotional crisis as the motivation to change our hairstyle completely. Sometimes this works out very well: you find that the new look suits you and the process of achieving it distracts you from your crisis. But all too often such impulsiveness ends in tragedy. In the heat of the moment, try not to rush out and get all your hair cut off. Don't get a permanent when the washing machine breaks. Don't become a blonde

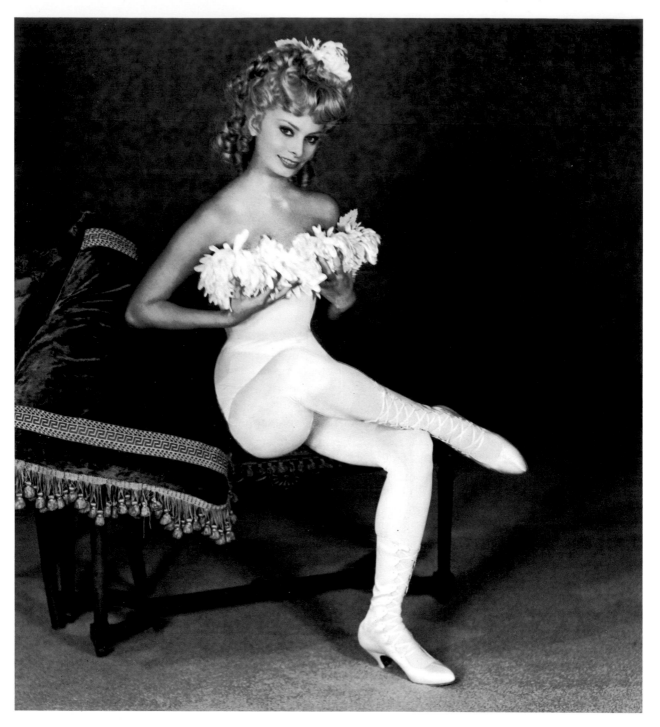

Here I am as a voluptuous blonde in Heller in Pink Tights, *1961.*

when you lose your job. It is possible that when you calm down you will regret your haste, and it will take a long time to get back to normal.

To be honest, I should tell you that I don't always follow my own advice. When I am in a crisis, I cut my bangs. As I worry, I snip away, and the shorter they get the more worried I become. At least, the damage is minimal: I have learned that bristles can be lived with. But if you feel a powerful inclination to call the hairdresser and become a new person, take my advice and count to ten first.

Your Hairstylist

It is worth the trouble it takes to find the right hair stylist because it can make such a difference in the way you look. You might find an unpretentious local salon that is willing to work with your hair and your schedule which is just right for you. Don't be misled by fancy salons. Just be certain of what you want – the results are what count. My stylist is Alexandre in Paris. I feel comfortable with him and I like the way he treats my hair.

Once you find a stylist you would like to try, I think it is a good idea first to make an appointment for a consultation. Make it clear that this is what you have in mind. It will only take a few minutes of the stylist's time, and it is a good way to learn if he or she is going to do the best possible job for you. Besides, once you are actually seated in the chair with a robe about your shoulders, you may find that reason deserts you. If the stylist wants to try something radical, you may have less resistance. But if you visit the salon beforehand, dressed in your street clothes, you will be in a more rational frame of mind. You will also have the advantage of being able to go home and think about it.

When you do find a stylist and are ready for a new look, think of the hair stylist as an educator, and ask a few important questions. How difficult will the style upkeep be? Is it a look that needs to be set every night? If so, is this something you can fit into your schedule? Is the style one that you can manage yourself at home?

I must admit that I don't enjoy spending time at a salon; I don't really like the ambience. Some women go to a salon to relax, but I would so much rather relax at home. A hairstyle shouldn't be a form of slavery, and it is very important to me to be able to handle my hair by myself.

Here is my daily hair routine. When I get up in the morning, I brush my hair carefully. Then, just using my fingertips, I lightly moisten the ends with water before setting my hair in a few rollers. After setting, I spray my hair with cologne. This is a trick that saves time as well as giving a lovely scent to my hair, for the alcohol in the cologne helps to dry the hair very quickly. Once my hair is set I put on my makeup, do some odds and ends, and then get dressed. By that time my hair is dry and ready to be combed out.

This brief set gives my hair a nice natural movement. I really don't like hair that is stiff with spray and looks like a helmet. My routine is easy and simple. I am quite comfortable doing it myself, and I will risk flattering myself by saying that I do a pretty good job. Of course, there are days when I am staying at home with the children or wearing a hat as a cover-up when I do next to nothing with my hair – just brush it and go. I suppose it is to Alexandre's credit that my cut is good enough to carry me through such days.

Color and Processing

Thinking of hair color reminds me of when I was very young and, like most young women, never content with the way I looked. I used to change my hair color almost every day – or at least it seemed that way. One day I would be a redhead, the next a blonde and finally a brunette. In 1954, when I was nineteen years old, I was filming *Lucky to Be a Woman* with Charles Boyer and Marcello Mastroianni. During the course of the film, I dyed my hair nearly every other day. I began as a brunette and ended it as a blonde. Fortunately, the film was in black and white, and I don't think anyone noticed! Sometimes professional obligations gave me an excuse for a quick change. Also in 1954, I made *Woman of the River* as a brunette, and a few weeks later I was filming *Too Bad She's Bad* as a blonde. I don't think there is any color that would be news to my hair.

But of course these were the excesses of youth and even now when I think about it, all that constant experimentation seems charming. Today my hair is just a bit lighter than my natural color. The lightness brightens my face and I am happy with it. When I am in Paris, Alexandre does it for me, but other times I can do it myself. If you have dark hair and want to lighten it, I recommend that you use subtle red or light brown highlights, as blond highlights look too harsh and fake.

If you are thinking of changing your hair color, consider carefully before you do anything. There are many very safe and gentle processes you can use, but a new color changes the texture and behavior of your hair, and you have to learn how to treat it differently. Perhaps more important, you have to be sure that the color looks right on you. I think that often it is a mistake to go from a very dark shade to a very light one. Most often the natural color of your complexion will not agree with such a drastic change. By the same token, a blonde with a very pale skin will find that a dark hair color looks unreal on her. It is very hard to make rules for what to expect, because each woman has individual color tones to her skin and hair, but I do recommend if you decide to change your hair color that you go to an expert the first time.

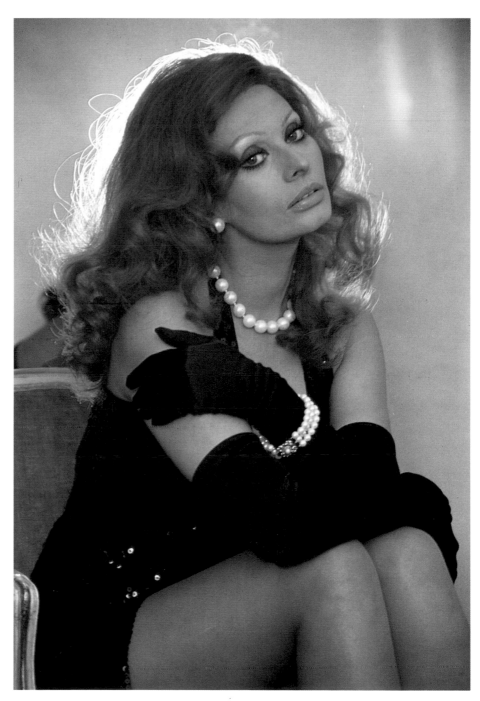

As the cabaret singer in Gun Moll *(1974) I was a redhead.*

One way to get an idea of how such a change will work for you is to try on wigs in a department store: ignore the style and just try to judge the effect that the color has on your complexion.

Another way you can dramatically change the look of your hair is to have a permanent. I have seen many women with perms who look wonderful, but my own experience was not so happy. Two years ago my hairdresser persuaded me to get one. After seeing all those magazine photographs of women with beautiful curls and inspiring "body" in their hair, I thought a permanent might be just the thing for my fine hair. What I didn't know is that with a permanent you have to give more care to your hair. The ends got quite dry and brittle. I also had to learn new ways of setting and caring for it. My hair became a sort of monster that needed to be pampered and coddled if I wanted it to behave. I was very relieved when it finally grew out and left me in peace. I don't think I will ever get a perm again. The purpose of my story is not to warn you away from perms but simply to tell you to be prepared for the new care your hair will need if you do decide to have one.

Cleansing and Conditioning Your Hair

Shampooing is the mainstay of hair care. It is the most frequent attention that you give your hair, and I believe that it is very important to shampoo often and correctly. No matter what your hairstyle, there is no reason to have hair that is less than perfectly clean.

In terms of oiliness, I suppose my hair is average and, as I've said, it is fine. I shampoo it three times a week. I am very careful to use a mild shampoo that won't damage my hair. I advise you to try different shampoos until you find one that leaves your hair shining and in good condition. I also think it is a good idea to change shampoos occasionally. After a few months any shampoo begins to lose its effectiveness, and it is time to switch to another for a while.

Be careful how you shampoo. Your hair should be completely wet before you apply a small amount of shampoo to the palm of your hand. Add some water to dilute it a bit. When you put the shampoo on your hair, massage it in very carefully – you can break your hair if you rub in the shampoo as though you are washing an old mop instead of fragile strands.

A hairdresser told me that many women ask what kind of shampoo their salon uses because they find their hair is especially clean after it has been washed there. The real reason for this, he said, is that the shampooer at the salon uses more care when washing hair than most women do at home. In his opinion, women need to shampoo more thoroughly and lather carefully, paying special attention to the hair near the scalp. Of course, you know that it is vital to rinse your hair thoroughly. Keep running warm water through it until every last bit of soap is gone and the hair squeaks.

I use a mild conditioner or cream rinse when I have finished shampooing, which allows me to comb my hair without breaking it. It also helps to make the hair manageable. You should experiment to find a conditioner that works for you and your hair type; some conditioners will make your hair too limp or greasy.

I might mention here that in winter if you find your hair becomes fly-away from the decreased humidity in the air, using a conditioner will prevent some static. It also helps to use a wide-toothed aluminum comb instead of the usual plastic one, but be sure that the ends of the teeth are smooth and rounded and won't tear your hair.

Wet hair is very vulnerable to breakage. Many otherwise careful women turn into demons after washing their hair. Even if you just pull at a tangle, the hair will break. It is best not to brush your hair at all when it is wet, but rather to comb it carefully. Brush it only after it has dried.

Every now and again you will need to use a deep conditioner on your hair. Perhaps because of my Italian heritage, I used to think that olive oil was the best conditioner, but if you don't like the idea there are plenty of oil conditioners on the market. An oil treatment is especially beneficial if you are spending some time in the sun. It protects your hair from drying out while at the same time conditioning it. Just comb the oil through your hair – you might want to warm it first if you are not going into the sun – and let it stay on your hair for a few hours. Then wash your hair thoroughly. You may have to use two or more soapings to get the oil and its scent out completely, but this treatment will give your hair a special luster.

THE SKIN AND ITS CARE

When I was in London filming *A Countess from Hong Kong*, I went to hear Barbra Streisand sing. I think her voice is very lovely, and I am a big fan of hers. After the concert I went backstage to congratulate her. The first thing I noticed was how beautiful her skin is – absolutely radiant and glowing. I couldn't resist touching it, and when I put my palm to her cheek I found it was as soft as my baby Edoardo's.

Even if you don't have a complexion like hers, you can easily improve what you do have. It is gratifying to take good care of your skin because it responds so quickly. And caring for it is an investment for the future, because a woman with lovely skin will look pretty no matter what her age.

I am lucky with my skin because it is what is termed "normal"; that is, it is neither dry nor oily. When I was a teenager I had an oily nose and I had to be careful to keep it especially clean so it wouldn't shine. To tell the truth, I think having oily skin as a teenager is a blessing, for it teaches you to care for your skin from an early age. Women with dry skin often have the most beautiful complexions when they are young, and they get spoiled. They don't realize that their good complexion is fleeting and that only constant moisturizing will keep it in condition. Another useful aspect about oily skin is that the film of oil retards wrinkles and your face ages less quickly.

The fact that skin changes over time is important, because if you are not aware of the changes, you can take the wrong approach to skin care. The most common mistake is for a woman who had oily skin as a teenager to continue to use strong cleansers and astringents on her face long after the oiliness has disappeared. She is really harming her complexion by drying out a skin that is already dry.

Skin – the Mirror of Health

It is amazing how quickly the state of your health shows up on your skin. The minute before you faint, for example, you become deathly pale and anyone looking at you knows that something is wrong. On the other hand, a pregnant woman's skin glows. I know that hormones play a big role in this radiance, but I also think that many women take better care of their health

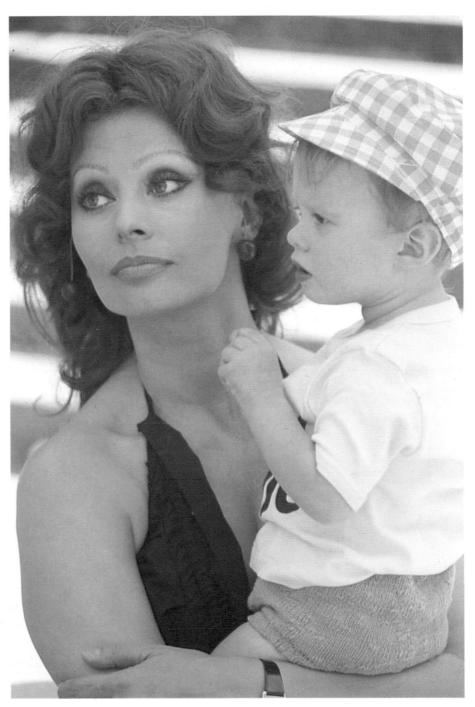

With Edoardo, 1974.

when they are waiting for a baby and this shows in their skin.

Your skin will never be at its best if your body is run down, if you don't get any exercise, if you drink and smoke too much, if your diet is bad. All these evils will show up on your face. Unfortunately, it takes some time for you to notice that your skin is deteriorating. Some people never make the connection between unhealthy skin and a bad diet, for example. It is too easy to think that you can just use more makeup or change your makeup techniques to cover up problems. However, if you live an unhealthy life, no makeup can disguise that fact.

Taking exercise is the best way of helping your skin. When you exercise enough to increase your heartbeat and therefore your circulation, you are helping the body clean the skin from the inside. After all, the blood washes impurities from the skin, but it can't do its job if your circulation is sluggish. Exercise will bring color to your face – that's the blood giving you an interior facial. The good effects last long after you stop exercising.

There is no doubt that drinking and smoking are bad for the skin; they both add impurities to the body which eventually show up on the face in the form of blotches, dryness, flakes and uneven color. Smoking not only damages your health, it also, in a purely mechanical way, makes your skin wrinkle, because when you smoke you purse your lips around the cigarette. Over the years tiny wrinkles form above and below your lips; lipstick runs into the wrinkles, and even if you are not wearing lipstick, the lines are still visible.

The biggest hazard to my skin is poker! I love to play poker, but when I do I stay up too late, am tempted to smoke, and eat things I would never consider in the cold light of day. Television provides the same temptation for some people: they find that smoking and eating TV snacks go hand in hand with watching a favorite show. Keep these inclinations in mind so you can avoid the source of the problem.

Of course, no woman is going to change her life for the sake of her skin. My point is simply to remind you that all these abuses are connected and they really will damage your skin. You can't expect to escape the ravages of time if you are the one doing the ravaging.

Water and Your Skin

It is easy to forget how important water is to the beauty of your complexion. Water, after all, is an essential component of skin. When your skin loses water, it becomes dry and tight. You feel as if you are wearing a dress that is a size too small. But when your skin is moist, it feels soft and supple.

Heat, especially dry indoor heat, is an enemy of soft, healthy skin because it draws out the moisture and is therefore drying and aging. Of course, you can add moisture to your face in the form of creams and lotions, but another trick I strongly recommend is adding humidity to the air. You can do this in several ways. Most simply, you can put containers of water near the heating source, or you can have plenty of plants which create humidity in the room. The best and most effective approach, however, is to buy humidifiers so that all the air in your house is moist. If you cannot afford one in every room, do at least have one in your bedroom.

I first learned about humidifiers when Carlo Jr. was a baby. Because infants are so susceptible to respiratory infections, the doctor recommended that I get a humidifier. He told me that when nasal passages and throats get dry, they can't fight invasions of germs; but moisture helps the body ward off these problems before they even begin. It seemed to me that if this helped Carlo it would be good for me too, so I bought one for my own room. Soon I noticed that my skin was much softer. And it is very nice to get fewer winter colds and sore throats. If you work in an office all day, it may well be worth humidifying the air there as well as in your home. If you don't feel like investing in a humidifier, put some plants in your office.

As well as making sure you have plenty of external moisture, you can also improve the look of your skin by drinking more water. The fluids that circulate in the body are keeping the skin clear by flushing away impurities. If you drink enough water – about eight glasses a day – this will help your skin stay clear and fresh. This liquid doesn't have to be plain water; it can also be in the form of fruit juice or mineral water or some form of tea or coffee (although you certainly shouldn't drink eight cups of coffee a day). I have a friend who indulges in all sorts of herb teas. She takes chamomile tea to soothe her nerves, peppermint tea to help digestion, rose-hip tea with Vitamin C to ward off colds. I don't know if these remedies really work, but she has beautiful skin and I think it is from drinking all that liquid. I rely on lots of mineral water with a slice of lemon or lime and sip it during the day to keep my skin fresh and dewy. My grandmother used to prepare for me a simple drink which I recommend highly: a glass of hot, sweetened water with a slice of lemon peel, which she called *canarino* because of its canary-yellow color.

Cleansing and Moisturizing Your Skin

Now we come to the pleasurable part of skin care: the cleansing and moisturizing ritual. This should be an important part of your day, not only because it makes you look better, but also because having a ritual, a sort of ceremony that is both relaxing and satisfying, makes you feel serene. It gives you time to let your mind wander and to refresh your spirits. The very action of smoothing cream on your face soothes as it releases tension and cares.

You must give your face a thorough cleansing at least twice a day: in the morning when you get up and at night before you go to bed. The only real difference in these two cleansings is the moisturizer that you apply afterward. At night you might use a heavier night cream, while after your morning cleansing you are probably going to make up and your moisturizer will be lighter.

I know that there is some controversy about the best way to clean one's face: some people swear by cleansing cream, others are devoted to soap and water. In my opinion, as long as you are meticulous about keeping your skin clean it doesn't matter which method you use. I have seen women with beautiful skin who use either method.

I use a cleansing cream on my face. The water in Europe is very hard and drying, so I tissue off the cream. When you apply a cleansing cream, or anything else, to your face, you should be careful always to use light, circular movements with your fingertips. If you rub with your hands, you will pull at the skin, stretch it this way and that, and eventually you will destroy some of its elasticity.

Sometimes in the morning after I have cleansed my face, I fill the basin with water and add a few ice cubes. Then I plunge my face into the cold water. This tightens the pores and I find it very good for my skin. It wakes me right up and makes my eyes clear and bright. Of course, if your skin is delicate, you must be careful not to use very cold water (or very hot, for that matter) on your face because such extremes of temperature can break the tiny veins on your face and you will have red lines that will be difficult to get rid of.

Many people find when they wake up in the morning that their eyes are a bit swollen. This is caused by water that collects in the tissues during the night. The puffiness will disappear on its own in an hour or so, but if you can't wait as long as that to put on makeup, try soaking two cotton balls in cold milk and put one on each eye for ten minutes or so. This treatment will quickly help your eyes get back to normal. A slice of cucumber on each eye will also do the trick.

Once I have cleansed my face, I put some Vitamin A cream under my eyes. I find that this is the best cream for me because others that I have tried are too oily. Also Vitamin A cream doesn't make the eyes swell and it doesn't promote an allergic reaction. I don't use this cream anywhere except just below my eyes where the skin is fine and tends to dryness.

Because my skin is not dry and because the cream cleanser I use isn't drying, I don't use moisturizer on my face after cleansing. If you do, remember that the job of the moisturizer is to hold in water that is already there, so it helps to have your face a bit moist before you put on any cream. Many women use spray bottles of mineral water for this purpose. Since the

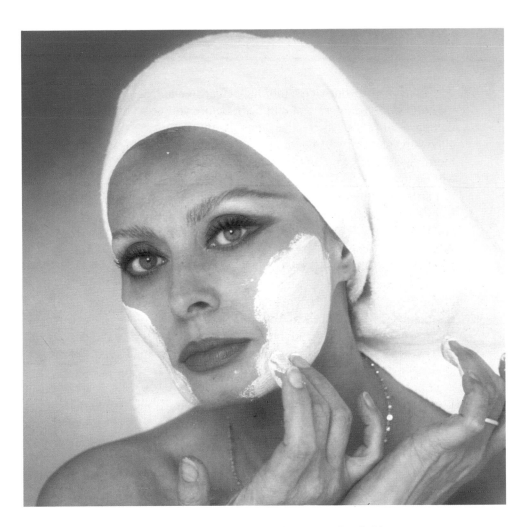

Giving yourself a facial is a special treat: it will remove dead skin and leave your complexion clean and soft.

Using a water spray not only tones and refreshes the skin but helps to retain moisture before you apply your make-up.

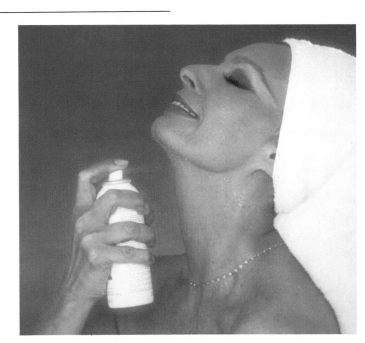

skin will not absorb thick, oily creams, they have no added benefit over a light moisturizing cream. Moreover, a thick cream is more likely to clog the pores.

As part of your cleansing ritual in the evening, be certain to remove all the eye makeup you have been wearing during the day. If you leave mascara on your lashes, this will dry them and make them brittle. And if you don't clean your eyes properly, you will have smudges on your pillow and will wake up with big rings around your eyes. Any kind of pure oil like baby oil or petroleum jelly is fine for taking off eye makeup; there is no need to spend a lot of money on creams that are made for the purpose. Just be careful that you don't pull the delicate skin under your eyes when you remove the oil.

Your Beauty Routine

There is more to skin care than just looking after your face. Your hands, feet and elbows need care, as does all the skin on your body. I am always impressed by soft feet and polished toes in sandals and by beautifully tended hands. These are the details of beauty care that can make all the difference.

You need to pay regular attention to the rough areas of your skin, and this takes some discipline. It is depressing to see how quickly the benefits of weeks of cuticle creaming or months of using pumice on your feet can disappear if you abandon your efforts. Regular care is a must.

I think the best way to ensure regular care is to create a spa in your own home. Some women have the time and money to go to commercial spas and that's wonderful. But it is only a brief experience, worth nothing if you don't continue with good care at home. I have never been to a spa other than the one I have at home because I am too self-conscious; I feel sure that people would recognize me and it would be difficult for me to benefit from the total relaxation that a spa should give. Having your own spa at home solves all those problems.

The hardest aspect of setting up a home spa is finding the time. There is always a claim on your attention. Nonetheless, it is important that you have time each week to take care of yourself. If you have a family, a good way to schedule your spa is to pick a night that features their favorite television show. You can make it clear to everyone that on that evening, during that show, you are not to be disturbed. Please do not feel guilty about doing this. On the contrary, it is a part of being a wife and mother to show your family that as a woman, you have an obligation to care for yourself and that it is a pleasure to do so.

Here are some of the things you will need for your spa. Gather them in advance so you don't have to run, dripping, from the bathroom.

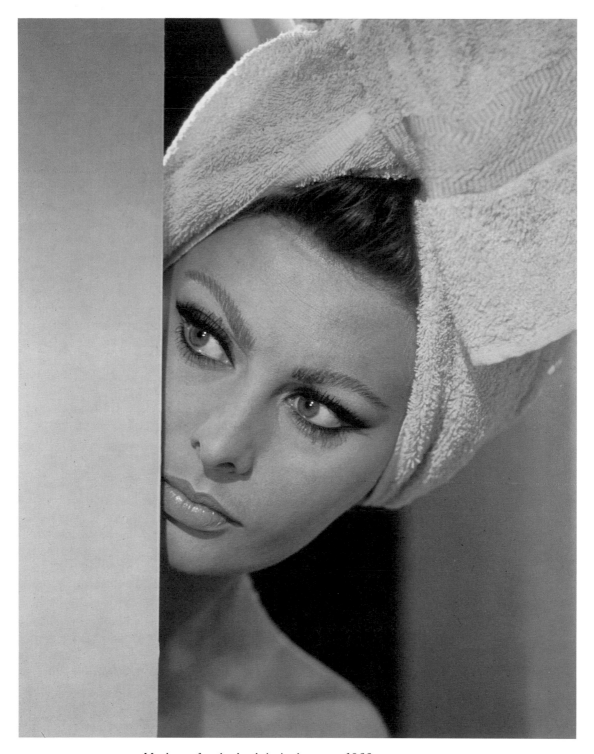

Made up for the bath in Arabesque, *1966.*

bath oil or bath salts
perfumed soap
dusting powder
body brush
pumice stone
facial masque
body lotion
razor and/or body-hair bleach
transistor radio

Here is a sample routine for a wonderful evening at your home spa. Begin with a few stretching exercises – the ones I have suggested on page 127 – to limber up your body and make you relaxed. Find some soothing music on the radio while you fill the bath, adding bath salts or oil. Meanwhile, steam your face briefly over the washbasin, using a towel on your head as a tent, then apply a facial masque. Get into the bathtub and relax, letting your mind wander. Use a pumice stone on your feet and heels and a body brush on the rest of you. Brush your nails with a nail brush and push back your cuticles with a washcloth. Shave your legs and under your arms. After your leisurely bath, take a quick, cool shower if you like, rinsing off the masque. Otherwise rinse off the masque in the washbasin after you are dry. Dry yourself with a thick, soft towel, and while you are still a bit damp put body lotion all over yourself and then dust yourself with powder. Now it is time for a manicure and pedicure.

By the end of your spa you will be ready for a glass of wine or a cup of tea. And you'll be irresistible!

The Bath

I love to take a bath using bath oil, perfumed soap and perfumed powder. One of the very nice things about having my own cosmetic line with Coty is that I now have all these products with a matching scent, my own "Sophia" perfume. By using them together when I bathe I can emphasize my perfume; and because it is a scent that I truly love, I like it to surround me all the time.

A bath is the core of your beauty routine. It relaxes you and softens your skin for any other treatment you might want to give it. But never allow the bathwater to become very hot. It is bad for your body to soak in hot water – it can even make you faint by raising your temperature too high. The ideal heat for a bath is just a few degrees above body temperature.

Part of the fun is adding something to the bathwater that smells good and helps your skin. In winter, putting milk in the bath will soften your skin and make you feel like Cleopatra. Using whole, fresh milk seems wasteful to me, but a cup of powdered instant milk will work just as well and is less expensive. In the summer it is nice to put some crushed mint leaves in your bath to make you feel fresh. I have read that the combination of mint and the herb marjoram added to the bath will calm nervousness. If you get sunburned, adding some apple-cider vinegar in the water will soothe your skin.

After you have let yourself relax thoroughly in the bath, you can go to work. While your skin is soft, use a pumice stone on your heels and elbows. I have been amazed to find how regular work on my feet can make them very soft. Once I got to the point where my feet became so rough they could rip stockings. But now, after constant attention, they are as soft as my children's. Your elbows and knees also need softening and you can lightly pumice them while you are in the bath, although what will really improve them is a good creaming afterward.

I also like to use a body brush on my body. It must be a very soft brush or it will irritate the skin. We have all heard so much about cellulite, that funny dimpled flesh that some women develop. The one thing I have heard that makes sense to me is that cellulite forms wherever blood circulation is not good. Using a body brush on those parts can stimulate circulation. I don't know if it really works, but it certainly won't do any harm.

Every other week or so I like to use a body peel. This is a cream that takes off the rough layers of skin, and it makes a big difference to the smoothness of my skin. Use it occasionally until your skin is as smooth as can be.

When your bath is over, be sure to put body lotion all over you. Because the body is warm and the pores are open, the lotion will absorb better than at any other time.

Facials

Giving yourself a facial is a special treat. There are many different types you can buy for different purposes. Once I had one that I would use before going out because it left my skin with a pink glow, which meant I could wear less makeup. I don't know whether any facials actually can change your complexion permanently, but they do help clean your skin and give it a rosy color.

Before you use a facial you should make sure your skin is very clean. You can clean your face by steaming, or simply use your everyday method of cleansing. I sometimes use a face peel that takes off the top layer of dead skin cells, but I do not use another facial after that because I feel it might irritate my skin. An old-fashioned way of freshening your skin is to use cornmeal. Mix yellow cornmeal with a cleansing cream to make a paste, then massage this paste over areas of your skin that tend to be oily – your nose, chin and forehead usually. Rinse and then put on an astringent. You

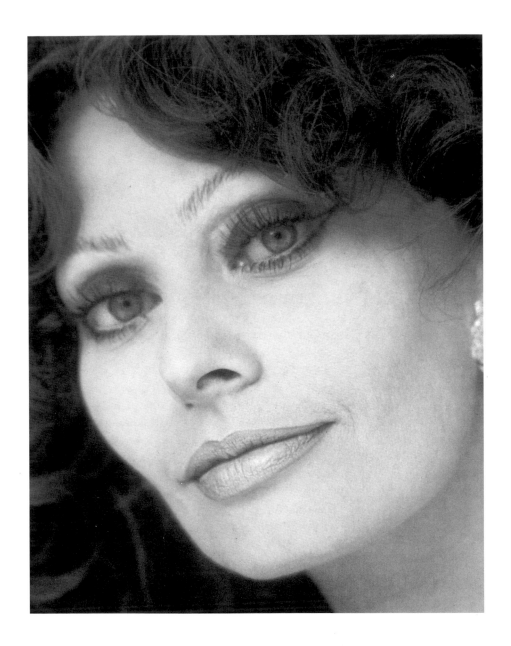

can follow the same procedure using sea salt mixed with mineral oil to form a paste. Both these treatments work the same way as a face peel to remove dead skin and soften your complexion.

Once your skin is clean you can apply a masque. There are so many on the market that you will find one that is just right for you. Or you can make your own masque by mixing oatmeal with water to make a paste. Apply the paste to your face in a thin layer, making sure to avoid the eye area. When it dries, wash it off with a washcloth. If your skin is dry, you can make a masque of powdered milk and water. Again, make a paste, apply it to your skin, let it dry, then wash it off. Your complexion will be clean and soft after these treatments.

Hand Care

Regular creaming is the best care for your hands, and if you do nothing else, this keeps them presentable. I have a bottle of hand cream near every washbasin and sink in the house. By creaming my hands after each washing, while they are still damp, I make certain they stay soft. I am also devoted to using rubber gloves when I wash dishes, but I have discovered that they have one disadvantage: because your hands are covered you think you can use water that is very, very hot. This hot water eventually harms your hands. So stick to your rubber gloves – fabric-lined ones are best – but don't use the hottest water. If you don't wear rubber gloves but must use soapy water, be sure to remove your rings first, since soap can collect under rings and irritate your skin.

I have never had the patience to have professional manicures. I prefer to look after my hands myself. Usually I file my nails just before I get into the bathtub. After I have soaked a bit and the water has softened my cuticles, I push them back with a washcloth or towel. I use a cuticle cream regularly – in fact I recommend that you have two or three little pots of it; keep one in your purse, in your car, near the phone, anywhere you are able to find a few minutes to rub the cream into your nails. It makes a dramatic difference to the condition of your cuticles and nails. I have very fragile nails and the cuticle cream has been a big help with this problem.

I don't use polish very often on my nails because I like the natural look. If you do wear polish remember that a light color makes your hands look longer and more graceful than dark red. A good trick is to add a spot of a bright-colored polish that you like to a bottle of clear polish. This will give a delicate tinge of color.

Here are a few more hand-care tips:

If, like me, you hate the smell that lingers on your hands after you slice onions, rub your hands with a little diluted cider vinegar, then wash them and you will find that the smell goes away.

Use a pencil or pen to dial the telephone. It saves your nails.

I used to love gardening in my villa in Marino, but I hated wearing gardening gloves as much as I hated getting my hands grimy. I learned that if you run your nails across a bar of soap before you

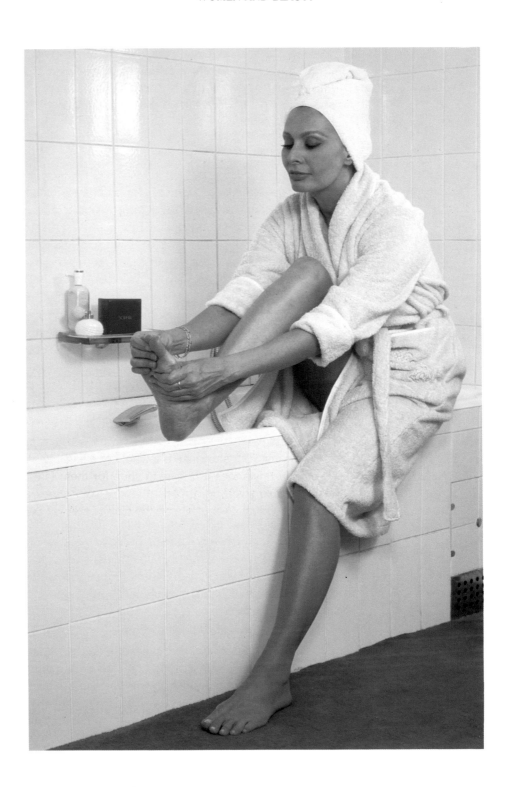

start digging in the ground, the soap will keep dirt from getting under your nails.

Cold winter air can chap your hands, so make a point of always wearing gloves. Rub in some hand cream before you put on your gloves, and by the time spring comes, your hands will be soft and pretty.

Foot Care

For me, feet are an erogenous zone. I love to have someone massage my feet, and I find that rolling my feet over a rolling pin while I am reading or watching television is relaxing. Eastern medicine holds that the feet are important because all the currents of energy in our bodies end there, and Orientals recommend that you make a point of massaging your feet when you get up in the morning.

If you have been using a pumice stone on your feet and also creaming them, the only other thing you have to do is give them a pedicure. I do mine in the bath unless I am putting on some polish. Sometimes I like to put polish on my toenails but I never use anything but a clear colorless one. Red toes are too bright for me; I think they look nice on many women, but I am not used to seeing that brightness at my feet. I like transparent polish because it looks as if you are pampered but it doesn't call attention to itself.

One thing to remember is that feet swell during the course of the day. You may find that your shoe size is a whole or a half size larger by dinnertime, so when you buy shoes it is best to shop for them late in the afternoon. Your feet will also swell on airplanes, and if your shoes are tight and you take them off, you may have to leave the plane barefoot! Swollen feet in stockings that are too small will develop ingrown toenails, so make sure your stockings extend a bit beyond your largest toe when you put them on in the morning.

Body Hair

There are a number of ways of removing excess body hair, but I have never done anything but shave. I do it in the bathtub using a fresh razor, and I am always careful to moisturize my skin afterward. It is wise to shave at the end of the day because after a night's sleep your skin is puffed up with fluids and you are more likely to nick yourself. If you do cut yourself while shaving, take a tip from men and use a styptic pencil to stop the bleeding. It is better than having those tiny pieces of tissue on your legs that you never remember to take off.

Another routine that I do as part of my home spa is bleach the hair on my arms. I don't really have much hair, but I like the look of smooth, soft arms. I use a solution of 10 percent peroxide mixed with a blond hair-coloring powder. I spread this on my arms and leave it on for about ten minutes, then wash it off. Not only does the solution lighten my hair so that it seems to disappear, it also smooths my arms by taking off the top layer of dead skin. When I have finished, my arms are very nice and soft. I do this about once a month, but your own schedule will depend on how dark your hair is and how fast it grows.

Maturing Skin

One of the biggest preoccupations we women have with our skin is how to keep it looking young. It seems that the goal of every cream, every complexion brush, every astringent is to make us look as if we had just wrapped ourselves in a brand-new mantle of skin fresh from our Maker. Oh, to have the skin of a child or, better still, a baby! Perhaps this is natural, yet sometimes it seems that we have become obsessive and really misdirected about our longing for a baby's skin. It is impossible to have young skin unless one is young.

I think a more satisfying and realistic approach to our quest for beautiful skin is to remember that the face is an indication of character. When we are young we are unformed, and there is little to see in our faces except the smoothness that nature has given them. However as time goes by, we take responsibility for our faces – not only in the care we give them but more important, in what they show of our natures. Boredom, complaints, bad temper, irritation are all visible in the face, and over a period of time become indelible. But serenity, humor, kindness and understanding also mark the face and will give it a timeless beauty.

I am not playing with words when I say this. It is really true. Look at the mature women you know and you can see for yourself. There comes a time when you don't notice wrinkles on a woman's face, you see only her character. Temperament begins to create a face when one is in the twenties, and by the age of fifty, a face owes more to its owner than to nature. So don't count your wrinkles and wring your hands. Be realistic about what you can do to improve your skin, but never compromise on improving your spirit.

Having understood that character is the most significant part of beauty, there is no reason not to do everything we can to enhance our physical gifts. There is much, for example, that we can and should do to slow down the aging of our skin.

Exaggerated facial expressions, for example, encourage lines and wrinkles that, with a little self-awareness, can be avoided. Many women frown constantly without realizing they are doing so. These frowns become

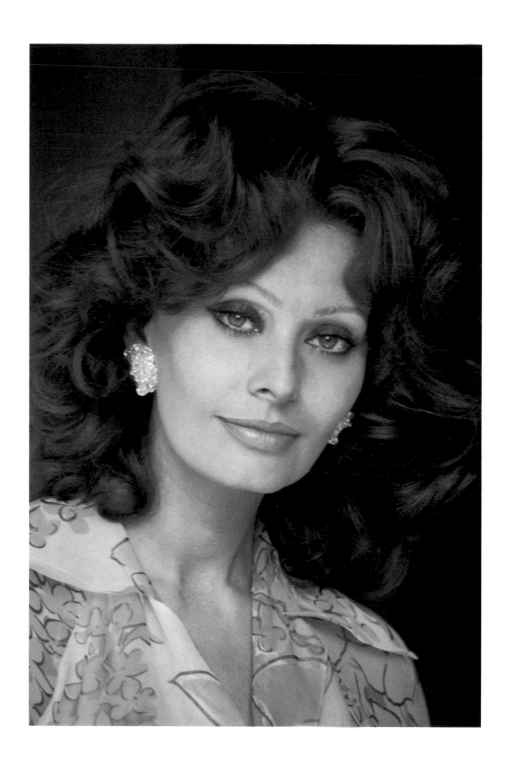

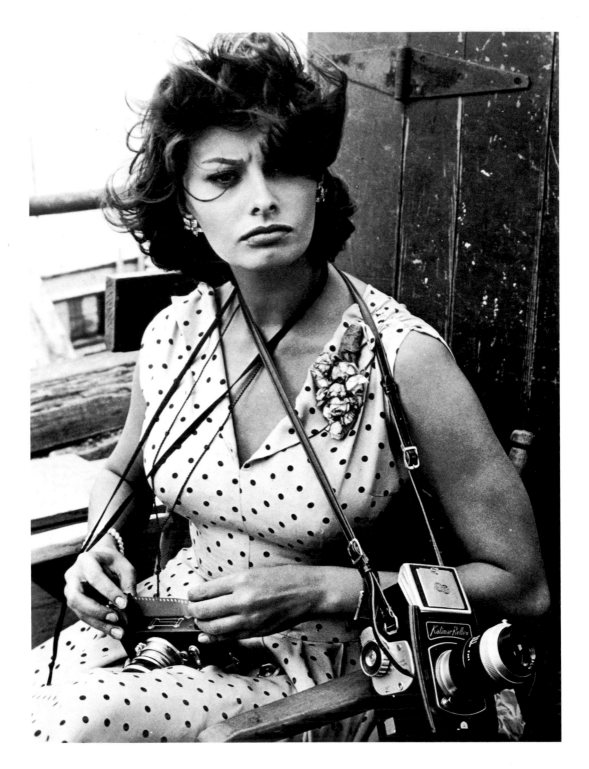

Frowning is a habit that we are often unaware of: here I am caught off-guard during the filming of That Kind of Woman, *1959.*

habitual and eventually their faces develop deep creases. I have an inventive writer friend who sits alone at a desk all day, and she told me about her unique solution to this problem. She puts a little piece of tape on her forehead or between her brows. Every time she begins to frown, she feels a tiny tug at her skin which reminds her to relax her face.

Try not to press your face hard into the pillow when you sleep, or get into the habit of sleeping facedown. Of course you will turn in your sleep, so make sure your pillow is soft, preferably of feathers. A foam rubber pillow gives more resistance, and after spending a night on one you are likely to wake with a face like a wrinkled prune.

If you are lucky enough to live in a sunny climate, you probably find that you are often squinting into the sun. Eventually lines will form around your eyes. Fortunately, this is easy to prevent. Just be sure that you always carry a pair of sunglasses to protect your eyes. It may be helpful to have more than one pair – keep one in your purse and another, for example, in the car. And don't forget that winter sun will make you squint as much as summer sun. If you are active out of doors in the winter, don't leave your sunglasses at home.

These little tricks are not worth becoming obsessive about, but if you can fit them into your life, they will prevent premature wrinkles and therefore are well worth the little bit of extra effort they take.

Tanning

The fashion for looking tanned began when I was a young girl. My sister Maria and I always longed for time to spend in the sun so we could have the bronzed look we associated with movie stars and the idle rich. One day we got our hands on a sun lamp and, filled with excitement, we set it up and prepared ourselves for a glorious tan. Talk about fool's gold! The instructions said that three minutes was the limit, but we couldn't believe we would get brown in that time, so we lingered under the lamp for what we thought was long enough. Afterward the two of us were riding in the backseat of a car while our mother, who knew nothing of our tanning adventure, drove. It was perhaps a half hour since we had turned off the lamp and we were anxiously waiting for our tans to blossom. Finally we began to get pink. A few miles later we were red; a few miles more and we were in agony, our faces swollen and the color of lobsters. All we could think about was what we would tell our mother when at last she turned around and saw us.

Despite that painful experience, I like to get tanned and I like to be in the sun. I think my skin looks very nice when it has a golden color. But one hears so much today about how bad the sun is for the skin, so I think one

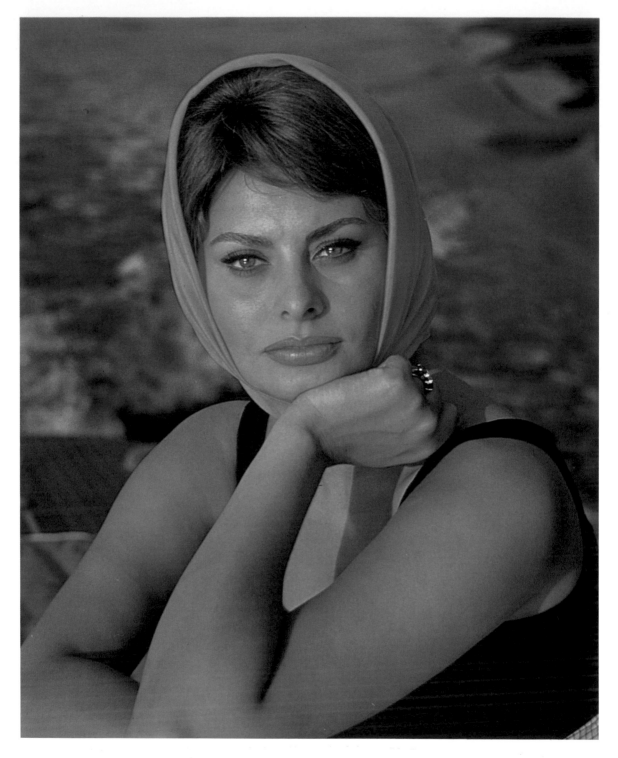

A golden tan like this always makes me feel really good.

must approach tanning with great care. First, you must know what kind of skin you have. I am lucky to have skin that tans easily; I don't have to sit for hours in the sun to get a nice color. Also I don't have a tendency to burn and my skin doesn't get dried out. But for women with fair skin or skin that burns easily, tanning is another story.

When I was filming *Woman of the River*, we were working south of Venice where the Po River meets the Adriatic Sea. The weather was beautiful and sunny. There was a production assistant on the set who had that wonderful pale porcelain skin of the north. Everyone warned her to stay out of the sun because her skin was so delicate, but she saw all of us enjoying the sun and she wouldn't listen. On the second day of filming she looked just like those red peppers you see in the market. The day after that, she was peeling terribly and it really hurt to look at her. I have never forgotten that girl because her sunburn was a vivid lesson in how the sun will treat everyone's skin differently, and you ignore those differences at your peril.

When the skin is burned by the sun it not only looks bad, it is actually damaged just as it is when burned by fire. When this happens over and over again, the skin loses its ability to recover. That is why women who live in very sunny places often have skin that is tough and leathery.

So if you want to have a tan, make sure that you never allow yourself to get burned. Today there are so many products to protect your skin from being sunburned that you should be able to spend as much time as you like in the sun. And there is no reason to be very dark – just a bit of color is fine. Fortunately, most women with delicate skin look best when they are pale or pink rather than any color the sun could give them. If they are going to be in the sun, they should preserve their delicate coloring and their skin's health by always wearing a sun block.

Before we leave the subject of tanning, I want to say something about those "tanning pills" you may have heard about. Called carotene pills, they are made from an extract that occurs naturally in carrots. They are supposed to make you tan, but in fact they just give you an odd orange color. I have seen people who take them all year long and they always look like boiled carrots. These pills are ineffective because you would never be fooled into thinking whoever takes them has a tan. So if you want to get a nice natural color, depend on the sun, not on pills.

THE ART OF MAKEUP

At the dressing table, every woman has a chance to be an artist, and art, as Aristotle said, "completes what nature left unfinished." As a makeup artist, you must remember that every work – every face – is unique. If you try to disguise yourself in order to approach an ideal, you will be making a mistake. You should be painting your own particular face so that whoever looks at it will have the joy of discovery as well as the joy of beauty.

Think of the irregularities of your face as the treasures they really are. Don't try to distort them. Dark stripes along your nose will not really make it look narrow, and lines that extend from the corners of your eyes will not increase their size. Concentrate instead on softening your extreme features so that they are seen as delightful peculiarities. Remember that a face with irregular features can be the mirror of a charming nature. Not only that, such a face is more memorable. Meryl Streep's nose gives her face strength and drama; without it, she would be diminished. When we see the character in her face, we know that this is a woman with confidence and spirit.

Faces in Fashion

If, like me, you have a strong nose or some other feature you think is less than perfect, there is another reason why you should make peace with it and learn to love it. Eventually it may become fashionable and then the world will love it too.

Once upon a time, when filmmakers tried to get me to shorten my nose, small noses were popular. The delicate noses of Grace Kelly and Audrey Hepburn were the standards to which all noses aspired. But times change. Today a strong nose is often considered an asset. Now no one would tell me to take off a bit of my nose as they did when I was starting out in films. Meryl Streep, Barbra Streisand and many other women with strong or irregular noses are considered beautiful.

There was a time when all women wanted tiny "bow" lips. The area all around the lips was covered with foundation and only the smallest curve of a lip, with all its fullness beneath the nose, was drawn in with a pencil. Today the sensuous mouth has come back into vogue.

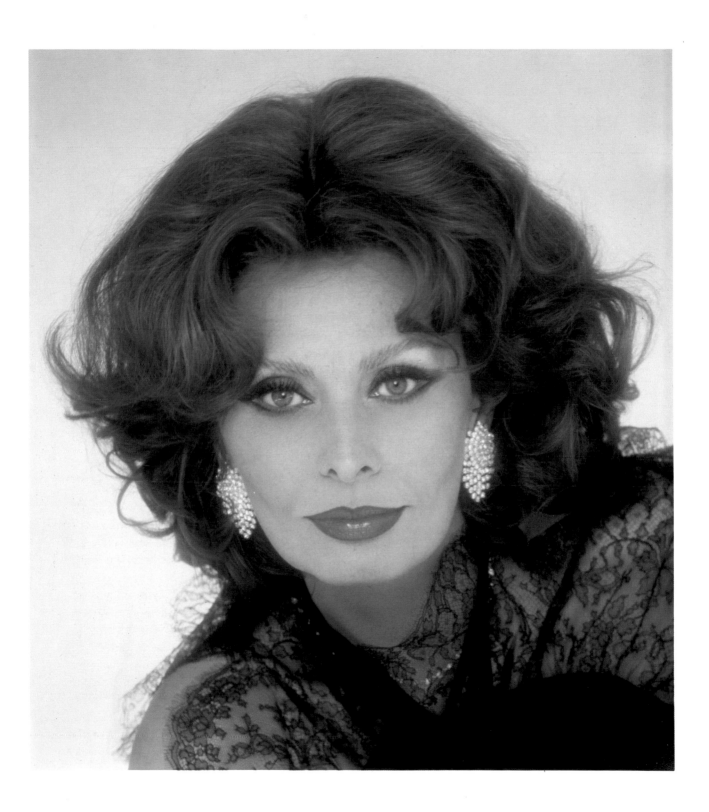

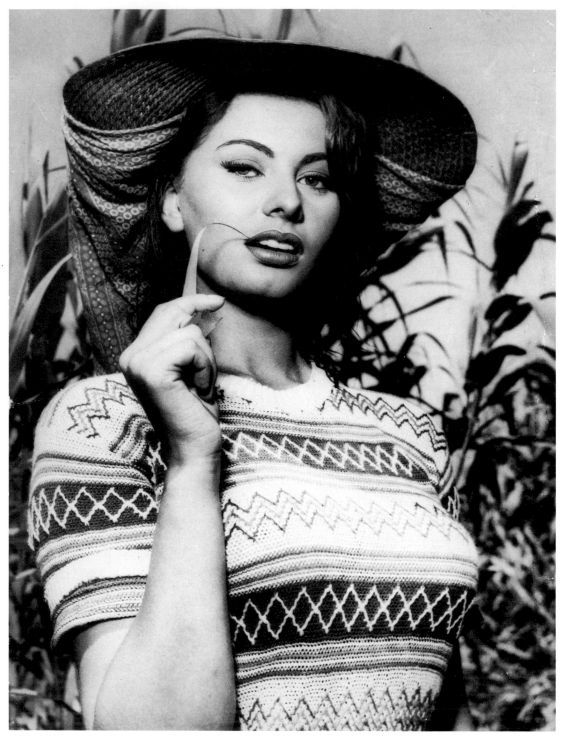

Here I am, not yet twenty years old, on the set of Woman of the River. *At this time plucked eyebrows were a must.*

Do you remember also the days of the thin, precise eyebrow? Some actresses, and many other women too, plucked out their eyebrows so that they could draw a fashionable line above their eyes. Unfortunately, many of these women discovered that their brows would never grow back: they had to draw in their brows forever. The lesson here is, if you have the strength to appreciate your idiosyncrasies, eventually the rest of the world will come to agree with you.

Knowing Your Own Face

Before you pick up your brushes, I would like to tell you one very important thing about makeup: only you can judge the effect of a technique on your own face. It does not matter if everyone tells you that the way to apply eye shadow is to blend it softly upward, or the way to use eyeliner is to put a thin line above your lashes. You may find that on your face, on your eyes, the way to use shadow or liner is different. I remember once seeeing a friend pluck the hairs on the top of her eyebrow. I told her I had heard many times that one was supposed only to pluck those that were below the brow. Well, she told me, she had always heard that too, but she much preferred the way her brows looked when she plucked them her own way. It makes you wonder who invents these "rules," and why.

I have spent hundreds of hours in the course of my film career having different makeup men and women work on me. I learned so many things from them! But now I no longer allow makeup people to work on me. I insist on doing it myself, for I feel that no one knows my face better than I do. I was beginning to find that each of the makeup artists had a different idea of how I should look. Sometimes it was very nice, sometimes not. But the big problem came when their idea of how I should look made me feel as if I were someone else. Then I would be very uncomfortable and my discomfort would show on my face. I felt like an impostor and behaved with the uneasiness of someone about to be caught committing a crime. This is a terrible state of mind for an actress, who needs to be relaxed and confident if she is going to be effective in her work. So now I just do it all myself and, for better or worse, I look like myself and no one else.

Although it is important to develop your own look, you shouldn't be inflexible in your makeup routines. Sometimes we grow accustomed to certain techniques that are no longer effective or are out of fashion. If I had continued with heavily made-up eyes, I would look like a woman who has not looked closely at herself since the late 1950s.

An excellent way to develop new techniques of making up is to go to department stores and experiment. When new items are being introduced, often there will be makeup experts to demonstrate products on you, and some department stores have special advisers there every day just to teach you how to apply makeup. If I hadn't already learned so much about it through my work as an actress, I would certainly take advantage of their expertise. Of course, you must be firm in your resolve to limit your purchases, or you may find yourself with a lifetime supply of products that you never use!

The Correct Light

Before you begin to apply your makeup, be sure that the light where you are working is right. If you are making up for daytime, you will get the best results working in daylight. Daylight is very harsh, and if you do your face in artificial light and then go outside, your makeup will look too obvious. Sometimes you will see a woman on her way to work in the morning, dressed very smartly but with two pink circles on her cheeks. These are a clear sign that she put on her makeup under dim light, probably in the bathroom under fluorescent lighting. If you make up in daylight, you will look fine under most other kinds of light. For this reason, when I travel I try to remember to take a portable mirror with me so that I can put on my makeup by the window instead of in a dimly lit bathroom. If you spend the day working under fluorescent lights, it is a good idea to keep a small hand mirror in your desk drawer. That way you can check your makeup to see if the tones are right. Remember that artificial light can change the color of blusher or lipstick; if they have a blue or brown cast, they will look dark and drab under fluorescent lights even if they look fine in daylight.

In most places in the world, the light in winter is different from summer light and you need to adjust your makeup accordingly. Pale winter light means that your face can do with more color to brighten it. In summer the light is warmer and you probably have more natural color, so you can use a lighter hand with your cheek color and eye makeup.

Daytime Makeup

My makeup routine is fairly simple. If I am staying at home with my family, I do the absolute minimum because I like to give my face a chance to breathe. I just use some moisturizer and a bit of color on my cheeks. But if I am going out, here is my daytime makeup procedure.

Foundation goes on first. The purpose of foundation is not to create a blank mask but to balance skin tones and conceal tiny imperfections. If my face is tanned, the sun has done the work of foundation and I skip it entirely. But when I am pale, I find a foundation is necessary. A light touch is best. In fact, as you get older, it is better to use less foundation rather than more,

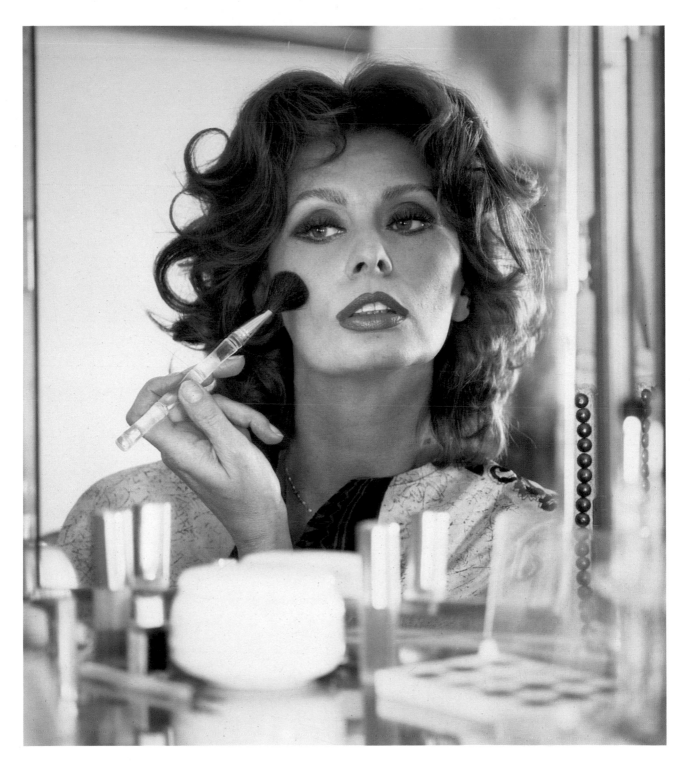

After I have put on my foundation I always buff it with a sponge and dust my face with a little powder to take away the shine.

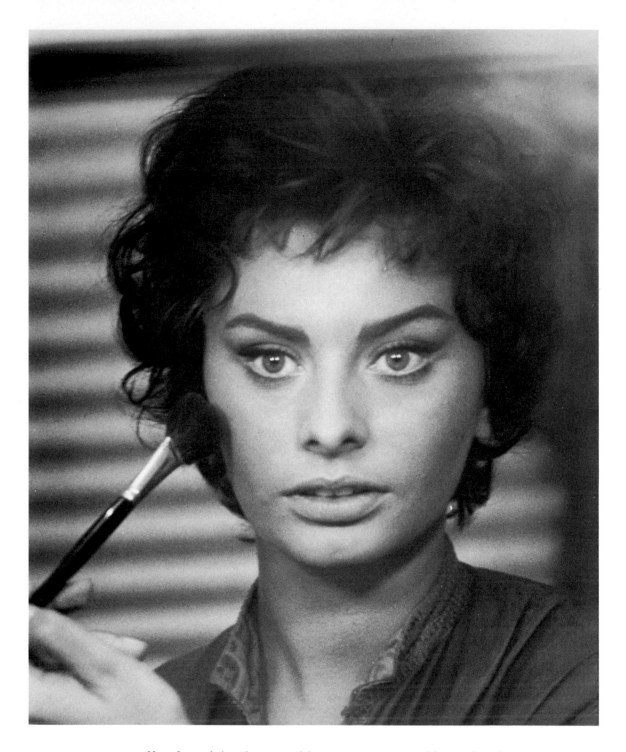

Here I am doing the same thing, many years ago. I learned early on that face powder is best applied with a big, soft makeup brush, as this achieves the most natural results.

although you may be tempted to increase the amount. Many women make the mistake of trying to conceal their years with thick foundation. But nature insists on the truth! If you use too much foundation, it will settle into any wrinkles and lines, emphasizing rather than disguising them.

I think the idea of putting foundation all over your face is old-fashioned; it is more effective to use it only where you need it. For most women, that means on the nose, the chin and perhaps the forehead. The goal is to tone down any heightened color so that it blends in with the overall tone of the face. The nose, for example, is often a bit redder than the rest of the face, and foundation will make it recede.

Finding the right foundation can make a world of difference to the effect of your makeup. When you shop for foundation, don't test the color on the back of your hand because the skin on your hand is different in texture and color from the skin on your face. Instead, put foundation on your fingertip and try it on the side of your cheek. You can even try another brand right next to it to compare the effect. Check the lighting in the store. If it is very pink or harsh, it will affect the look of the foundation and its color.

Most bottled foundations are too drying for my skin. I use my own mixture of cream foundation in a tube plus a very dark stick makeup. I stroke the stick into my palm, and then squeeze a little of the cream foundation on top of it. I mix them with my finger until I get the right color. Then I use a sponge to apply the foundation to my face, stroking it on in an outward direction. By the way, if you have fine hair on your face, as many women do, a moisturized foundation with a dewy rather than a matte finish will look better. Apply the foundation in the direction of the hair growth and it will be smoother on the skin. If you want to make your foundation lighter and more moist, mix a tiny bit of your favorite moisturizer into it in the palm of your hand before you put it on.

After I have applied the foundation, I use a clean makeup sponge to buff it. This takes off most of the foundation, leaving just enough to give a soft, polished finish. Buffing in this way makes the foundation very subtle and natural-looking.

Finally, I dust a bit of powder on my face to set the foundation and take away any shine. Then I am ready to start on my eyes.

The Eyes

It is said that the eyes are an actor's most powerful tool because they have direct emotional control over an audience. If you watch great actors and actresses, you will notice that most of them have an intensity of expression in their eyes. Richard Burton is an example of someone who can hypnotize you with his eyes.

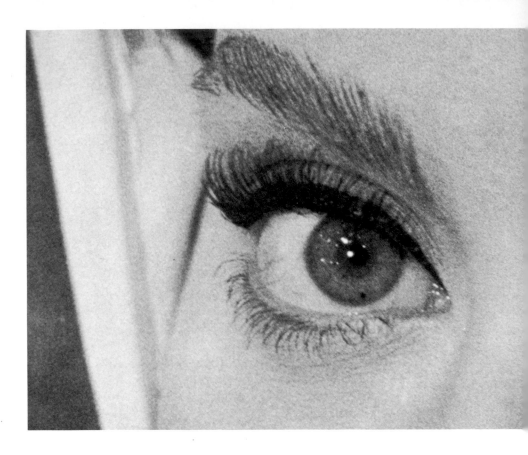

An actress's eyes are her most direct link with her audience.

Because the eyes are so powerful, I think they deserve the most attention when you use makeup. But attention does not mean exaggeration. When I see photographs of myself in the dramatic eye makeup of the past, I don't like it, although at the time I was accustomed to it. I think also perhaps I played up my eyes to distract attention from my nose, which was supposed to be too big.

The exaggeration of the eyes began in the mid-fifties with Audrey Hepburn. She had beautiful, large, gazelle-like eyes which she would emphasize with heavy makeup. She was so popular that everyone wanted to look like her, and so it became the fashion to have heavily made-up eyes. When the film *Cleopatra* came out in 1963, people were so amazed and enchanted by Elizabeth Taylor's exotic kohl-laden eyes that over-emphasized eyes became routine. I am glad that the style has changed and today a softer, more natural look is in fashion; for most women it is far more flattering.

The biggest challenge for me in doing my eyes was finding a makeup that would stay in place. Like many women, I have eyelids that tend to be greasy, and most makeup I used on my lids soon creased and faded. Eventually I

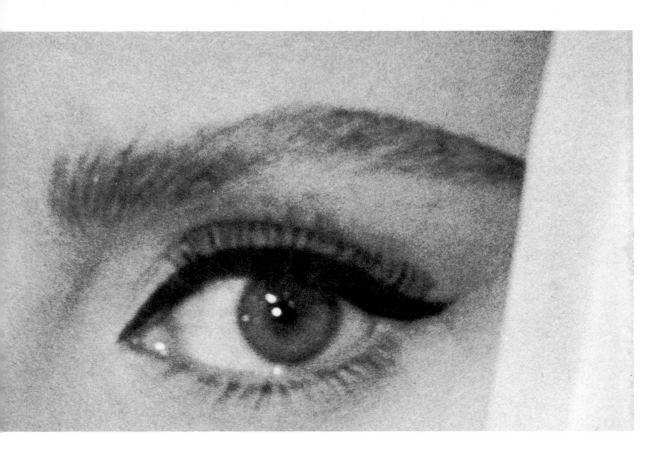

discovered that a liquid makeup would stay in place, and I use this as both a shadow and a liner. I prefer a very dark brown, nearly black shade, although I vary and soften the color by adding water. Diluted and applied with a medium brush, this liquid eye makeup works like shadow. Using it with little or no water gives a stronger color and when applied with a fine brush, it works as a liner just above my top lashes and below my bottom ones.

I learned how to make up my eyes from professionals. Every woman must learn for herself what technique works best for her. I discovered that my eyes look their best when I use a dark neutral color, blending it upward from above my lashes. I put the darkest color right above the lashes, lightening it as I move toward the natural crease above my eye.

By the way, if you use a light-colored concealer under your eyes, as I do occasionally, be very careful about the color. If it is too pale, you are in danger of looking like a raccoon! The shade must be just right – a tiny bit lighter than your foundation color. Also be careful how you apply the concealer. The skin beneath your eyes is the most delicate on your face, and this is one of the first areas to show age. The skin is very thin and constantly in motion as you blink, smile, frown and laugh. Treat it gently by patting on the concealer with your fingertips. I think it is wise to avoid stick concealers as they pull the skin too much; use a cream instead. Be sure to blend the concealer carefully so that it disappears into your foundation. If you have trouble making the concealer look natural, try putting it just below the circles under your eyes instead of directly beneath the eyes themselves. This is often more effective.

After I have finished with the liner and shadow, it is time to put on mascara, which I apply with a lavish hand. Black mascara gives my eyes the great intensity that I love. If you are a blonde with very light lashes and brows, you might prefer brown mascara, but most women look better in black. I put on several coats of mascara, but I am always careful to let each coat dry, and then I brush it out so the lashes don't clump into spikes. You can buy tiny combs for that very purpose.

If you use mascara that comes in a little cylinder with its own brush, you will probably find that when you first open it, the mascara is too wet and thick to do a good job. A friend told me that to solve this problem she always lets a new mascara sit open for a few days before she uses it. It gets a bit dried out and works much better.

Eyebrows are the frame of the eyes. I use an eyebrow pencil to adjust mine, although I always follow the natural line closely. If I want to seem a little more assertive, I use more pencil; when my mood is sweet and gentle, just a feathery brush of pencil does the trick. I use a brown pencil and make tiny strokes to look as if they were really hairs. A heavy painted line above the eyes doesn't look right – it's too overpowering – but little strokes can give more strength to weak brows or those that need a slight correction in their shape. If your eyebrows are wild, you may find that brushing on a little bit of lip gloss or hairstyling gel with an old toothbrush will help keep them in place.

Makeup Under Glasses

Making up your eyes when you wear glasses takes a bit of practice. If you are far-sighted like I am, the lenses magnify your eyes so you have to use a light, careful touch. Keep your makeup soft and muted and try to avoid harsh lines. Your eyeliner, if you use it, should be smudged a bit for the most natural look. Stay away from bright colors; neutrals are best. You might even find that if you use a powder blusher on your cheeks, a bit of that brushed over your lids and beneath your brow can be flattering. Be sure that you brush out your lashes carefully after your mascara goes on, because any beads or clumps will be magnified. Your eyebrows too should be neatly plucked and in place – I always use lip gloss on mine to hold them.

If you are near-sighted, you must take the opposite approach. Because your glasses minimize your eyes, you must emphasize them. Eyeliner can be very helpful. Stick to a neutral shade for the liner and your eye shadow. You can afford to put on more shadow than a far-sighted woman, and you might

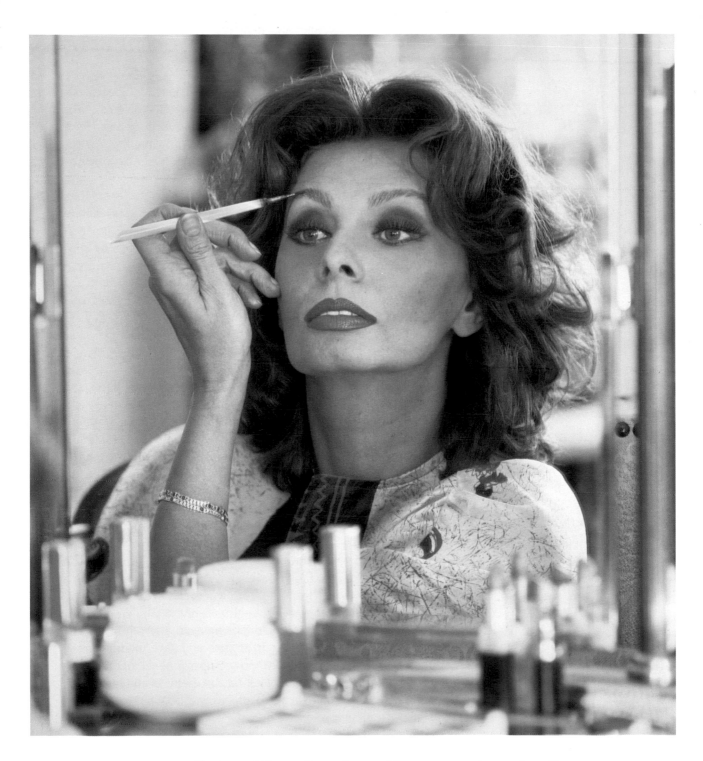

Try to avoid heavy lines when making up your eyebrows. I use tiny pencil strokes, following carefully the natural line of the brow.

also want to use a light-colored shadow below your brow and above your lashes to highlight your eyes. If your brows are light, use a pencil to make them stronger, but don't use a very dark color – it will only look strange. If your brows are exceptionally pale, you might consider having them dyed, but never try to do this yourself because it is too dangerous; find a beauty salon that will do it for you.

A woman who wears glasses should apply her blusher only after she has got her glasses on; otherwise any cheek color that is under the glass will be affected by the lens and might look exaggerated. After you have finished making up your eyes, put on your glasses and check everything to be sure that the emphasis and the colors are right.

The Reds

When the foundation and the eyes are finished, it is time for the reds – the lips and cheeks. Red is passion and fire. I love wearing red, and I think that what red can do for the spirit it can do for the face. Perhaps it is as simple as the connection between blood and the color red which makes us think of it as passionate and bold. So when you come to the lips and the cheeks, you have a chance to express a little passion – with subtlety, of course.

I have found with my lips that the passion I express must be smoldering rather than a roaring fire! I can't wear emphatic bright or deep reds because if I do, all people can see then is lips. The color of lipstick that you can wear depends on your skin tones. When I use a lipstick that has any purple in it, my lips, which are already dark, become terribly exaggerated.

I found my perfect lipstick color about twenty years ago. It is a mix of pink and beige that is somewhat light and somehow perfect on my lips. Fortunately, it also goes with most of my clothes. I fell in love with this lipstick and wore it all the time. Then about seven years ago I was searching for it and discovered that I was living on borrowed time: my favorite color was no longer being manufactured. Fortunately, I had a friend who was working for the company that had made that lipstick. She found all the leftover lipsticks in my shade that were in storage and gave them to me. I now have about ten left. What I will do when they are gone, I can't tell you, but I imagine the solution will demand great resourcefulness and flexibility. In the meantime I am storing them in a cool place away from the light so that they will last as long as possible.

Sometimes I have to change my lipstick when I am wearing an outfit that clashes with my usual color. Before you put on lipstick you should be careful to check the shade with your clothes. I don't think it is necessary to fuss too much about matching clothes with makeup, but there are colors – some reds and oranges, for example – that really don't go together. Most

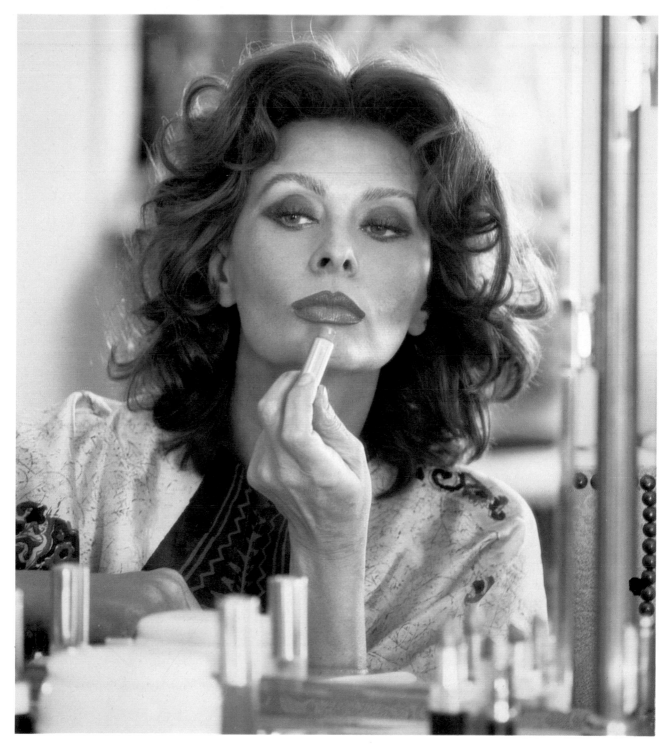

Again, I follow the natural curve of my lips when applying lipstick, outlining them in a slightly brighter shade.

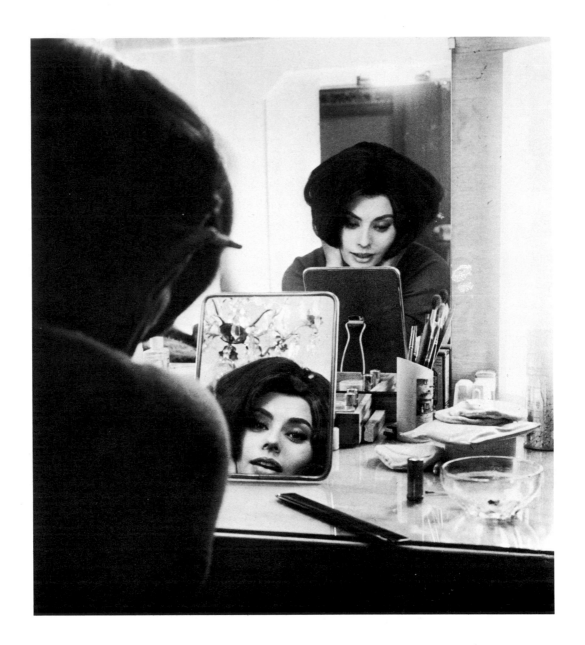

*Because I know my face as no makeup artist can, I am happier
doing my own makeup for my films.*

people have a color palette that they work with for both their clothes and their makeup, so things usually work out naturally.

I apply my lipstick in the usual way – straight from the holder. I don't use a lipstick brush, but I do sometimes outline my lips with a pencil that is a bit brighter than the lipstick itself. I follow the natural line of my lips whether or not I am using a pencil. My lips are certainly generous, but I don't see any reason to try to minimize them with lipstick techniques.

When most women think about lipstick, they imagine a closed mouth that looks soft and inviting, and forget that their lipstick color has to work with the shade of their teeth. This may sound fussy until you notice a woman with bright red lipstick and yellow teeth. There are lots of variations in tooth colors – just ask your dentist if you don't believe me. If your teeth have a yellowish tone, you should avoid lipsticks that are in the red-purple range and stick to the corals and red-oranges. The simplest thing to do is smile when you try on a new lipstick. Not only will you get an accurate idea of how the color will affect your teeth, you might also cheer up the salesperson behind the counter!

When I tell you how I give color to my cheeks you will understand how desperate I will be when my special lipstick is all gone. You see, I often use it to color my cheeks. I like them to have a bit of a shine, so I often take my lipstick and just gloss it over the top of my cheekbones. It gives me enough color and blends perfectly with my foundation and, of course, with my lipstick. Sometimes I add a bit of another color to make my cheeks brighter or darker. When I have a tan I find no need to add much color at all.

I know there are many rules about how to choose the right color for your cheeks according to your skin tones. I suggest, however, that on your next trip to buy makeup you cast aside all those rules and try a few shades of red that you never thought of before, just for fun. In my experience, most women get very set in their ways about the shade they wear on their cheeks: it's pink from sixteen to sixty and beyond, and a rose or a tawny red is never considered. But you might be surprised to find that a change in color gives your face a real lift. It is worth a try, and the worst that can happen is that when you leave the store, you look like a little girl who invaded her mother's dressing table and went wild!

In general, powder blush adheres better to dry skin, while gel color lasts longer on oily skin. Some modern gels and powders are intended to give a sun-kissed look. I have never tried them, but a friend tells me that they work very well if you put the color in the places where the sun would hit your face: on the top of your forehead, the tops of your cheeks, along your nose and on your chin. The color should be light and well blended. My friend uses this technique when she goes on vacation to a warm climate; the extra color saves her from that pale newcomer look of the first two days.

Makeup for Evening

In the evening some of the makeup rules change. The mood shifts: sometimes you will want to dazzle, sometimes seduce. In any case you will want to look your best, whether for a large crowd at a party or for the one person in your life who matters the most. I am more playful, more dramatic and more amusing with my evening makeup. I am never really extreme, but more willing to try something unusual. Let your imagination go when you makeup for evening, but be careful not to go over the top. You don't want to look ridiculous, you want to look special.

The first consideration when making up for the evening is lighting. For me this is especially important because if I am going to be in a public place and there will be photographers, I have to be very subtle in my makeup. This is because flash bulbs are like daylight, and if my makeup is heavy I look like a clown in photographs. In most cases evening light will be softer and more flattering than daylight. Whether it is candlelight or the soft light of a restaurant or dinner party, it allows you greater freedom to use deeper colors and more extravagant flourishes. You can add more color to your cheeks, a deeper shade on your eyes and more mascara and lipstick. Evening is the only time I use a colored eye shadow, for example. During the day I stick to neutral tones, but at night I can put a bit of a color on my eyes and it will look fine.

One of the reasons your makeup should be more dramatic in the evening is that you are usually wearing clothes that are different from the business-like wardrobe of the day. If you are wearing jewels or even simple costume jewelry, your makeup has to stand up to them; your face should not disappear in the sparkle of earrings and necklace. And if you are wearing an elegant dress, your face should be in harmony. When a woman dresses for the evening but wears daytime makeup, it looks to me as if she is just trying on the dress, not really wearing it.

Evening makeup provides a great opportunity to realize a fantasy. It encourages us all to become actresses. The woman who spends the day in a business suit with just a bit of mascara and lipstick on her face can become a gypsy at night with smoldering eyes and ruby lips. The nurse can become a princess, the mother a sophisticate. The opportunities are unlimited. This element of fantasy is important to every woman and should not be ignored. The evening is no time for the timid and the ordinary. Even if you don't sparkle with witty conversation, you can still sparkle with makeup that tells the world you are a woman of mystery and surprise.

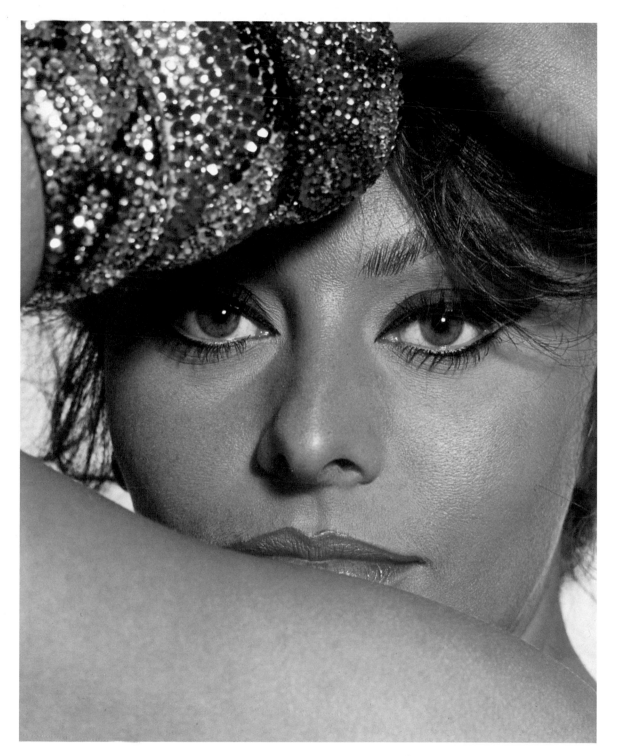

When you are as tanned as this, you can afford to wear less makeup.

FASHION AND A SENSE OF STYLE

*T*ry to imagine what it might be like to be a child dressed always in hand-me-down clothes, with the nickname of "Stuzzicadente" (toothpick) and the feeling that you had your face pressed up to the window of life. Then suddenly, or so it seems, you are a creature besieged by journalists, working with the most glamorous men of your time and participating in a life of amazing luxury.

Looking back on the child I was, my life seems a fairytale. Certainly I have been fortunate. But my point in describing the circumstances of my childhood is not to arouse sympathy – I am grateful for the experience of poverty – but to show you what a large leap it was suddenly to find myself attending fashionable parties, meeting famous people and traveling in a world that just a few years before was as foreign to me as life on the moon.

As you can imagine, I had a great deal to learn about fashion. When you understand the contrast between my youth and my early success, you will appreciate that I came to the world of sophisticated fashion a complete novice, and everything I learned, I had to pick up from experience and observation. I am not a fashion expert by any means, but I have come a long way. (Any woman who could wear the clothes by Dior in *Arabesque* and the Balmain fashions in *The Millionairess* and not learn something about style, would indeed be dull!) So I am happy to pass on to you the things that I had to learn the hard way.

The Journey to Simplicity

When I was a child of ten or eleven, my idea of a well-dressed woman was Rita Hayworth or Dorothy Lamour in a glamorous evening dress, sparkling with jewels and draped in fur. To my eyes, this was as beautiful as a woman could possibly be. But when I started to work in Rome at around fourteen, I had to face reality. I could no more buy an evening dress than fly. I simply didn't have the money to spend on clothes. Jewels and furs were things to dream about. Still, I needed to wear something appropriate when I met people and auditioned for work. So I discovered, by necessity, that simplicity is at the heart of elegance. I forgot this lesson for a while when I

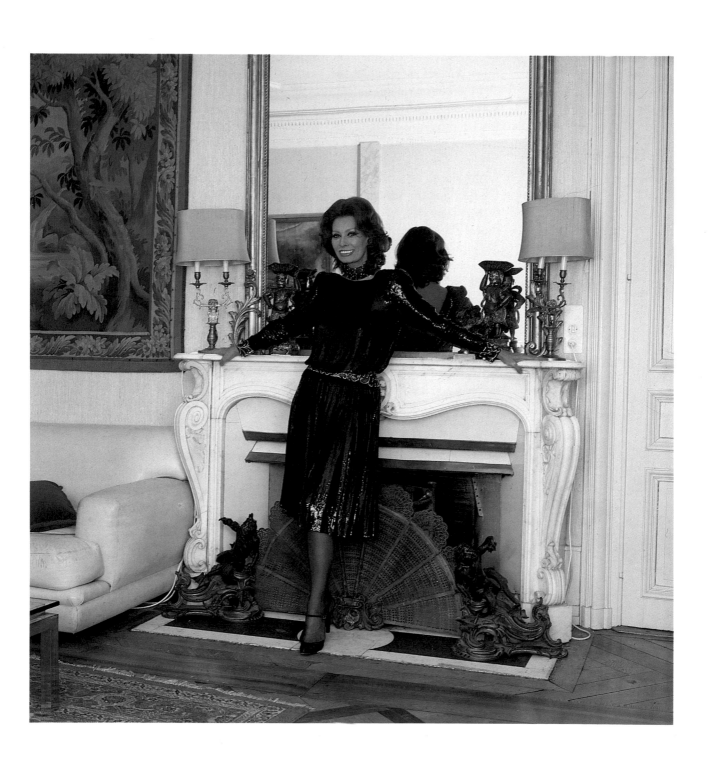

became very successful, but I remembered it later and I live by it today. I think it is the most valuable lesson a woman can learn about fashion.

In order to have something to wear in those early days in Rome, something that would cost practically nothing and could be worn all day long and into the evening, and on every sort of occasion, I took my clothes, my navy skirt and white blouse, and dyed them black. Even my handkerchief became black. It was the only way I could think of to provide a versatile wardrobe at no cost. And it worked. I could go anywhere in my black clothes, and the simplicity of my appearance was very elegant. Even when I was surrounded by women in expensive colorful dresses, I always felt comfortable in my black outfit. You may have noticed that a woman who is slightly underdressed often seems confident and relaxed. I wasn't aware of this when I was young, but I am now. It was really luck that my solution in black was tasteful. I only knew that it worked for me.

Later, when I became successful, I abandoned my simple, black dyed clothes and lived out the dreams of my youth. I bought fabulous evening gowns. I loved furs, especially ones with long hair like fox. And I bought a Cadillac in a very light blue color; for me, that is what it meant to be a star. If you are from a poor background, it takes a long time to learn that even though you may have the money to buy whatever you want, you don't have to flaunt your wealth. You don't have to wear jewels and furs to look elegant and successful.

Though in my case the change from poverty to wealth was extreme, I think the value of simplicity is something every woman should learn. In the last fifteen years I have found that what is simple and comfortable is usually best. It is not a matter of trying to control oneself, but more a gradual understanding of what is truly attractive.

I learned other, more particular things about fashion from acting in films. When you see yourself on screen, you are forced to recognize what suits you and what doesn't. You have instantly before you the image of yourself as you look to others. The camera is so critical – much more so than the naked eye – and it makes clear your defects right away. If you are not wearing the right shoes, the right makeup or the right clothes, it is apparent immediately.

After all my varied experience with clothes, I have come to the conclusion that elegance and style are really the best goals of fashion. They are the ideals that can guide you in your choice and help you find a look that is right for you and classically beautiful.

Elegance

To me, "elegance" in fashion means the classic tradition of timeless beauty and grace.

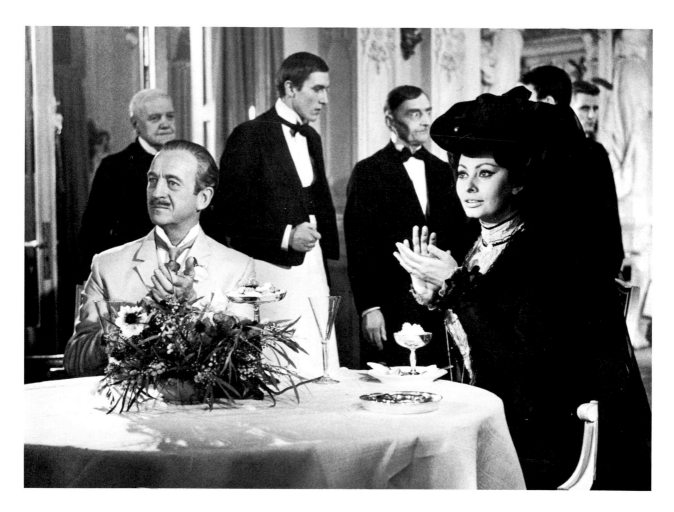

A taste of high living – as the elegant widowed countess in Lady L, *with David Niven, 1965.*

If you want to see if this definition of elegance really exists, I have a suggestion. Find an old fashion magazine – it may be two years or ten years or even twenty years old. As you thumb through the pages, many of the fashions will seem strange and even funny. You will see skirts so full that they look like whole bolts of cloth cut into circles, exaggerated shoulders and wildly varying skirt lengths. But you will find that some of the clothes stand out in a different way. They would look elegant if at that moment the model stepped out of the magazine and on to the street. These clothes usually follow some sort of classic line. (The Chanel suit is the best known example of this.) Because these fashions please the eye as much today as they did years ago, they are truly elegant.

Perhaps it takes a mature person to prefer elegance in fashion. My niece used to wear clothes that I found bizarre – baggy pants and strange tops that made her look like a farmer at harvest time. But if I said anything to her she would respond with, "Well, why do you dress like an old lady?" This transformation was natural. I didn't begin to dress "like an old lady" all of a sudden. When you are young you want to try everything. You wear clothes that after a few months are out of fashion. You wear any colors, any exciting combinations. You are eager to experiment and usually happy to follow the crowd. Eventually you begin to find a look that suits you. When finally you are mature, and surely there are some very young women who are quite mature about fashion, you realize that a timeless look is really the prime goal. This is when you are ready to appreciate elegance.

Thinking about timelessness reminds me of that most elegant of men, Cary Grant. In so many ways he is the ideal of elegance. Tall and slim, he moves in a naturally graceful way. Of course, there aren't many men who have the face of Cary Grant. But, as far as fashion is concerned, I can tell you that he is wearing the same clothes he wore when I first met him working on *The Pride and the Passion* in 1956. Well, perhaps he has bought a new suit or sweater since then! But he was the first man I ever saw sporting those unlined summer jackets and that wonderful blue-and-white pinstriped look that you see everywhere today. His appearance has a timeless quality.

Elegant fashion is always comfortable. The neckline that is too low, the waist that is too narrow, the hat that is so large it is about to fly down the street on a breeze – these are not elegant. Grace in movement is a large part of elegance and of course you won't be graceful if you are grappling with a sleeve that is falling off your shoulder or a skirt in which you can't walk. The most appealing example of elegance and comfort I can think of is the outfit Tony Asquith wore while he directed *The Millionairess.* Tony is the essence of a refined man: articulate, well educated and always gentle and considerate, he was a pleasure to work with. As a director he was on the go all day, and throughout the filming he wore the same faded blue-denim

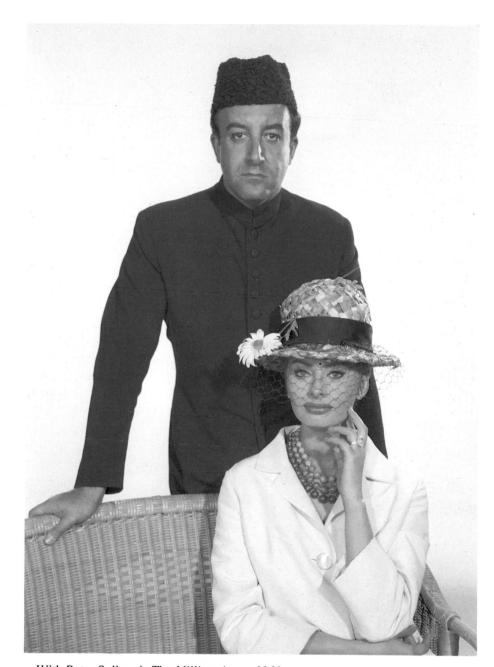

With Peter Sellers in The Millionairess, *1960.*

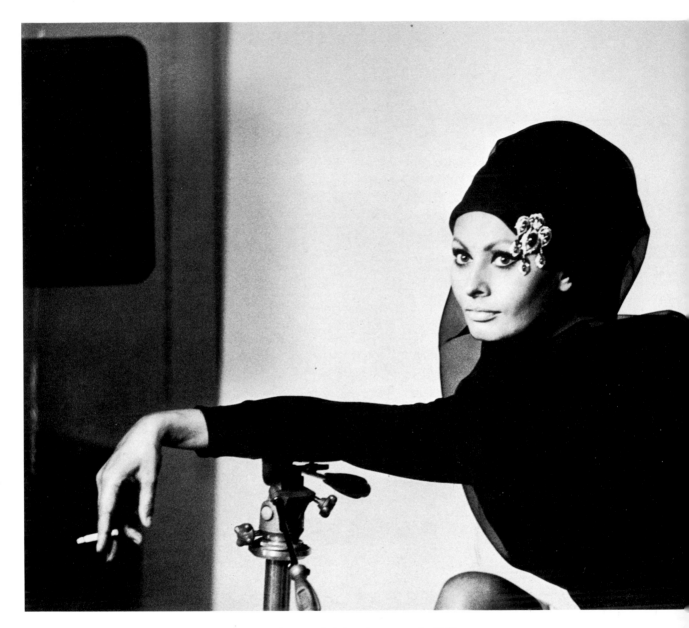

Dressed to kill for a publicity photograph, 1969.

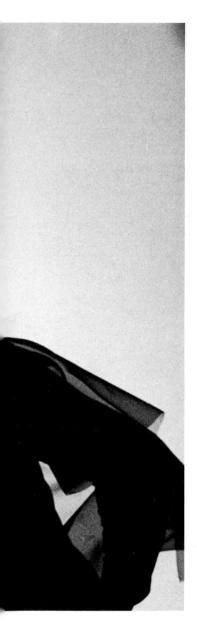

overalls. It was really an odd contrast – the gentleman in the worker's clothes – but I have never seen a man look more comfortably elegant.

Jean Cocteau, the French writer and poet, once said that "Elegance is the art of not astonishing." This applies to fashion as much as anything else. Grace Kelly epitomized a certain regal elegance that was never overshadowed by her clothes. She was never astonishing, always supremely elegant. The jewels and furs I once bought may have been luxurious, but they weren't always elegant. Elegance speaks softly. It has more to do with harmony than sensation. Perhaps when I wore a simple black dress with my dyed black handkerchief, I was more elegant than I could ever be in a fox fur. But this is a lesson that comes with time, and learning it is one of the pleasures of maturity.

Style

Style is the very personal accent that you give to your clothes to express yourself.

If elegance is about harmony, style is about individuality. Take for instance Elizabeth Taylor or Barbra Streisand. The way they dress could not be described as conventionally elegant, yet they both have a unique sense of how they want to look and a very personal style that goes beyond fashion. A woman with style is one who chooses the best that is available to her and then adds her own unique touch to make it special. If you have style, then you know how to take a trend or a fashion and personalize it. Some women do it with a hat or a scarf or an unexpected way of wearing a piece of jewelry. Style can be whimsical and fun. It can be anything that expresses your personality. Sometimes you can achieve a stylish look with a clever juxtaposition: perhaps a luxurious silk blouse worn with blue jeans.

Style cannot be bought. Some people are born with it; others develop it. In any case it does not depend on great expense. We have all seen the shopgirl on her way to work wearing a charming cotton dress with a scarf tied just so and a jaunty hat that completes the look. That is style.

Some Fashion Guidelines

Style and elegance are so difficult to define exactly. Yet we all know them when we see them. One thing is crucial if you want to achieve style and elegance: attention to detail.

I am not suggesting that you must spend long hours examining your wardrobe and shopping. I am encouraging you to consider carefully before you buy anything. Explore wearing different combinations of clothes you already have. Think about everything you put on. You don't have to match

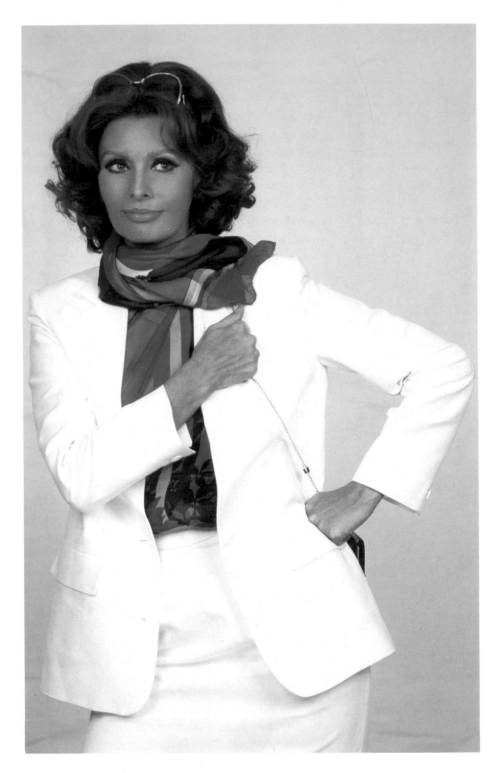

A timeless, classical look that will take you anywhere.

things in a conventional way, but you have to know how they work together. Sometimes attention to detail means removing some of your jewelry because it is excessive or adding a small brooch on your coat lapel for a bit of color. Sometimes it means wearing less makeup or a more simple hairstyle. I have a friend who usually wears her long hair tied back, but instead of a rubber band she uses colorful ribbons. Such small things make a great difference.

As we all know so well, fashion is always changing. Coco Chanel once said, "Fashion is that thing which is soon out of fashion." Remember the miniskirt or the peasant look? Something very much in style today may look ridiculous tomorrow. If this is true, how can you achieve a look of timeless elegance? Should you ignore fashion entirely?

There are four "permanent" considerations you should make before you buy anything. If you think about each of them and how they apply to your own life, then you will be better prepared each time you shop. Gradually they will become almost unconscious guidelines that will keep you from making the wrong purchases. I should admit that I am not a great planner when it comes to my wardrobe, but I do try to think about these four points before I buy something. They are: quality, life-style, color and self-expression.

Quality

If you want to achieve an elegant look, you must develop an eye for quality.

Quality does not mean that a garment must be expensive. It means that the fabric, the cut, the construction, the color and the line should be as good as you can afford. Before you buy something, check the seams, make sure the patterns match and that the fabric has a "feel" you like. Clothing that is poorly made, of inferior material, no matter how expensive, will not flatter you and will not last. You will be so much better off buying clothes that are of the best quality, not only because they will last longer, but also because you will feel good each time you wear them. I once bought a pair of simple, tailored black slacks that I felt were too expensive, but they fitted so well I couldn't resist them. Gradually they became my favorites because each time I put them on I felt terrific, and they were worth every penny I had spent on them because I wore them long after I had discarded cheaper clothes.

Today the influence of excellent designers is felt all over the world. Manufacturers seem finally to have learned that inexpensive clothing doesn't have to look cheap. You don't have to be rich to buy quality items. Of course, some clothes are wildly expensive – in fact, sometimes when I look at the prices in fashion magazines, it is hard to believe that people can afford to buy them. It is one thing to spend a lot of money on an elaborate evening gown, but how can you justify a breathtaking price for a simple shirt or sweater? Still, if you shop very carefully and with an educated eye, you will be able to find clothing that will make you look elegant and stylish for a long time.

A good way to learn about quality is to visit the most expensive store in your area. Though not all the clothes you see will be first rate, many of them will be. You do not have to buy anything, just look around. Don't let the sales helps intimidate you; they are there to help. Feel the fabrics, take note of the colors and try on the clothes that please you. This will help you develop an eye for excellence.

Here is one last tip on shopping for quality. I think that one of the biggest mistakes women make when buying clothes is buying them a bit too tight. If you examine couture fashions or look at magazine photographs of models dressed in expensive clothes, you will notice that these women are rarely wearing tight garments. There is a generosity of cut to quality clothing. The goal is always to give a fabric its own line and flow. In tight clothes the fabric never moves; this is the hallmark of cheap fashions. Next time you buy slacks or a dress or a blouse, look for a generous cut to the material and don't try to squeeze into a size that will impress no one but the cashier who sees the label.

Life-style

Today we women lead very complicated lives. We are at home, we work in offices, we run errands in the car, we care for children, we cook – often all in the same day! We need clothes that are comfortable, look nonchalant and are easy to wear.

Spend your fashion budget where you spend your time: if you are in an office most of the week, then office clothing should take the lion's share of your clothes budget. Many women fall into the trap of spending a great deal of money on an evening or a "dress up" wardrobe that they wear only a few hours a month or even a year. This is fantasy dressing. If you don't often wear formal clothes, then don't spend a great deal of money on them. Or find one wonderful, versatile evening outfit that is expensive but will last you for years and years.

I buy couture clothes because I need them for professional occasions. Twice a year I go and select some new items for my wardrobe, and I concentrate on those dress designers who have the ability to make outfits that are elegant but nonchalant. It is very hard to find clothes that combine these qualities.

No matter where you buy your clothes, let me remind you that you have to be firm about what you really like and what you think looks good on you. We

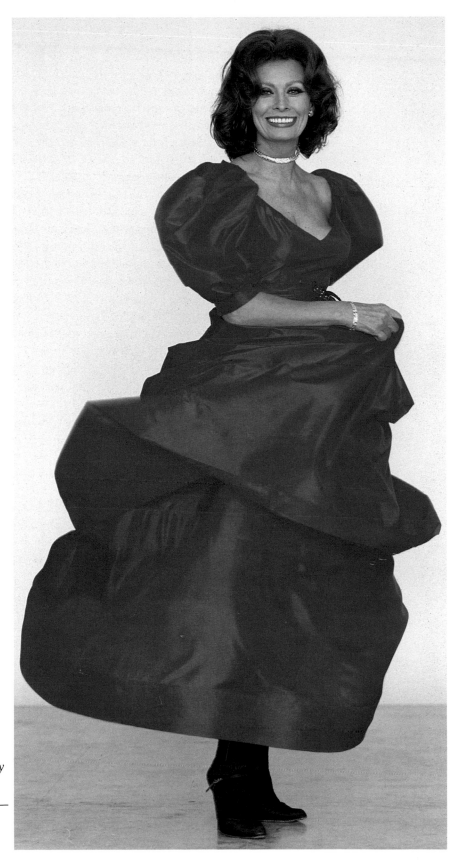

I like clothes that allow for plenty of movement.

sometimes make our worst shopping mistakes at the prompting of someone who doesn't share our precise taste. I remember when Balmain made a beautiful red dress for me that I loved on the hanger but hated on me. It was tight and I hate tight clothes. Even though he, and other people, said they loved the way the dress looked on me, I never felt at home in it. Much to his dismay, I could never bring myself to wear it.

If your day is spent at home, you should spend your money on attractive casual clothes. Don't just slip into jeans every single day because "no one will see me." This is bad for morale. Jeans are very nice – I wear them often – but not as a steady diet. Invest in some simple, stylish items that you will feel happy to put on in the morning and that will take you through a busy day. I have recently discovered how comfortable and versatile running suits can be. I have some in four bright colors, and if I am going to be at home all day, doing chores around the house, that is when I wear them. Like jeans, they shouldn't be overdone, but they are hard to beat on a busy morning when you are rushing to get the kids off to school.

Remember also that you should make an effort to look attractive in the evening for the man in your life, even if you are only going to be watching television together. It is very tempting to come home from a busy day and change into an old bathrobe. If this is the type of garment you like to wear in the evening, buy yourself an elegant one; you will feel so much better that it will make your evenings more pleasant. Once when I was in the Far East, I found some very beautiful silk material that I brought home and had made into caftans. I wore these caftans all the time at home, even to sleep in, and because I hate wearing clothes that are tight, I especially loved their flowing lines. They turned out to be a really good investment because I got so much wear out of them and they always made me feel attractive, even if I was just cooking dinner. I think it is important to have some casual clothes that are very pretty as well as being comfortable.

Color

Most women eventually find that there are a few colors that are flattering to them and they tend to buy them over and over again. I am one of those people. I think this is perfectly fine, and if you do the same thing, you will probably find, like me, that every now and again you'll be tempted to buy something in another shade. You will get tired of looking always at the same things that catch your eye in the store because they are "your" color. It is good to experiment and perhaps you will find a new color that suits you. But don't be led astray by salespeople who want to sell you something pink because everything is in pink that year. You alone know best what is right for you.

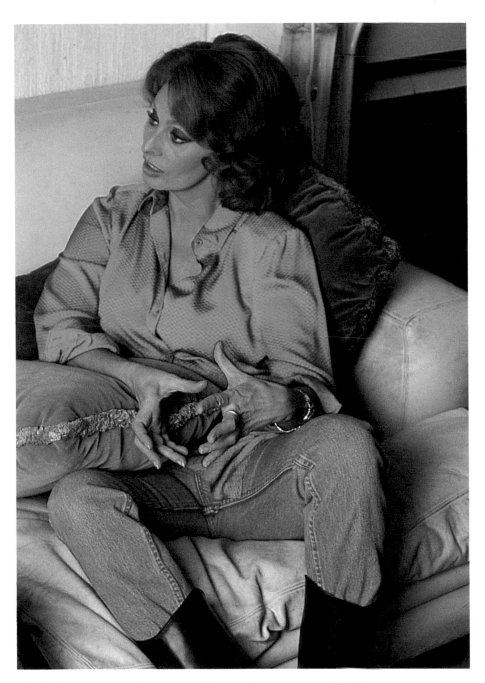

Blue jeans worn with a smart shirt and boots can be effective.

Here's a tip to keep in mind for deciding on colors when you are buying clothes: make sure that you are wearing the right makeup. Some colors that don't look good on you when you are wearing minimal makeup might be very flattering otherwise. I learned this on the movie set when sometimes I had to wear costumes in colors I thought would look awful on me. Sure enough, when I tried on the costumes without first putting on makeup, they did look pretty awful. But once I had put on foundation, blusher and eye makeup, the colors became balanced somehow and looked fine. This is especially true with colors in the red family. The red sweater you try on with no makeup might make you look pale and wan, but with a brighter face it could be terrific.

As you know, black is one of my best colors. I brighten up my black clothes with a colorful scarf, but I find that I always feel confident and elegant in black. I also discovered by watching myself on the screen that red and white are flattering. Simple, bold colors seem to suit me best.

Purple is the only shade I never wear except as an occasional accent. It is too violent a color for me. Moreover, in Italy there is a superstition among actors that purple is bad luck. I don't really believe this, but I also think I might as well not tempt fate! I remember how Vittorio de Sica hated the color purple. While we were shooting *Lady L* in the Nice studios, I was living at the Negresco Hotel in Nice. The Negresco has a salon with everything covered in purple velvet. When De Sica arrived in town, he came to visit me and they showed him to the purple salon. He was horrified, and when at last I found him he was on the other side of the hotel recovering from his bout with purple.

If you are unsure about colors, experiment but also ask your friends for reactions. Sometimes it is hard to judge for yourself how much difference a color can make. Don't forget that if you change your hair color or get a tan, the clothing colors that flatter you will change. And as you get older, your skin usually changes in tone; the navy blue that was wonderful when you were twenty might make you look too drab when you are forty.

One thing is certain: neutral colors are always elegant. Likewise, it is usually safer to select solid colors than prints. Prints are more difficult to harmonize and can look cheap if they are not in good taste. This is not a rule – you will sometimes find beautiful print fabrics – but it is something to keep in mind.

Once you find the colors that flatter you, stick with them. Of course, you will want to experiment with new ones and try different shades as accents. But it is so convenient, once you know what palette suits you, to choose all your clothes in those colors. Not only will you save time on shopping and avoid making errors, but you will find that there is more harmony in your wardrobe.

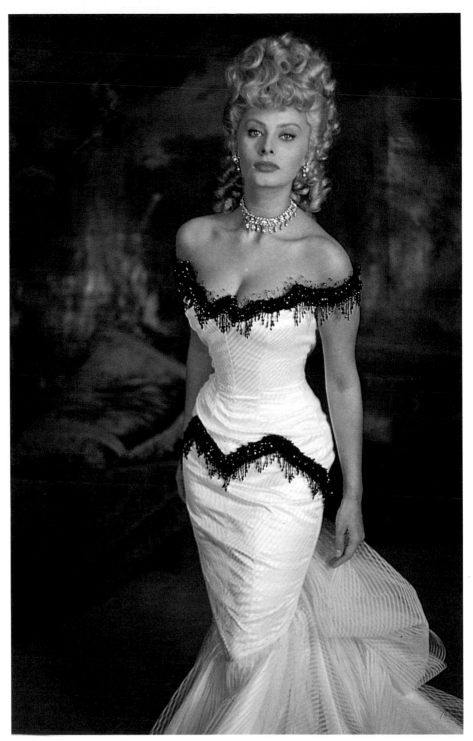

I came to like white after seeing myself in it on the screen – here in
Heller in Pink Tights.

Self-expression

Clothes are one of the most immediate means of communication. When you see a woman in running shorts, sneakers and a T-shirt, you know something about her without even talking to her. If you see a woman in a tailored suit, wearing a smart hat, and carrying a briefcase, you make certain assumptions about her. Jane Fonda and Dolly Parton each have their unique way of dressing, and even if you knew nothing about either of them, when you passed them on the street you would have some idea of their personalities just by looking at their clothes.

We all use fashion to tell the world something about ourselves and it is important to be aware of what that personal message is and whether it is accurate. Sometimes women can be unintentionally provocative or severe in their dress. This will affect not only the world's reaction to them but also their self-image and self-confidence. I once saw a woman at a party dressed in a flaming red dress slit to the thigh. Her neckline was breathtaking. This would have been all right if the woman had been up to it, but she wasn't. She spent the evening wondering how to handle the reactions she got and feeling very uncomfortable.

Self-expression should be fun. It is an opportunity to be creative and whimsical. It can be such a pleasure to express your moods through your clothes, sometimes complementing, sometimes offsetting them. If you feel depressed, a cheerful outfit can make the world manageable again. If you are feeling romantic, a beautiful soft blouse or flowing dress or robe can highlight your mood and make you feel like a heartbreaker. Once a friend gave me a pair of bright red knee socks; they had nautical symbols embroidered down the sides. Every time I put them on I felt cheerful because they were so amusing.

Self-expression is very much connected with style. It is your own way of showing the world what is unique about you. It is also a way of varying your wardrobe. You might have a single dress in a neutral color that you love. You wear it during the day with just a scarf at the neck and a leather belt and you feel comfortable. At night you can leave off the scarf and belt, add a necklace and earrings, and in your same comfortable dress you are now ready to go out to dinner. Another time if you are feeling very *au courant,* you can add a flamboyant bracelet or gypsy earrings and still feel comfortable but this time also a bit daring.

The Perfect Wardrobe

Most of us have a fantasy of the ideal wardrobe. In this dream, let's say you open a closet – a huge walk-in closet – and thousands of expensive blouses, sweaters, jackets and dresses greet your eye. Each item is exquisite and fits like a dream. Instead of having two or three favorite things to wear, you own about a thousand, with shoes to match. You have so many clothes that when you dress, instead of choosing a garment on the basis of what is clean and what is ironed, you simply indulge your mood. A sexy sheath dress for lunch with an old boyfriend. A flowered cotton jumper to collect the children from school. A silk caftan and sparkling jewels for an evening at home. I know how you feel because I have had this fantasy too. I have also had the opportunity to live it, and now I can tell you the truth about it.

If I could give you only one piece of advice about fashion it would be to forget the fantasy of the limitless closet and adopt instead the idea of the small but perfect wardrobe. Most of us are too greedy in our approach to clothes, and it leads us to feel perpetually dissatisfied because we believe that in order to be truly happy, we need more. A far better approach is to assume that there is a limit to the number of outfits you can use. Decide on what you *really* need and buy the best.

Have your basics of the finest possible quality, replace them when worn, and indulge yourself with accessories. A woman who takes this approach will always be well dressed, will always look elegant and sophisticated, will spend less time in despair in front of her closet, and will save both effort and money. Resolve right now to stop thinking about more clothes and start thinking about your own small, perfect wardrobe.

Shopping for Clothes

I confess that I don't like shopping for clothes. But I do enjoy having nice things to wear – indeed, I need them for my professional life as well as for home wear. So I have become very scientific about shopping. Unless you love shopping and have lots of time to spare, it is well worth developing your own "scientific" approach.

I used to buy clothes on impulse. Something in a store would catch my fancy. I would try it on and if I liked it, home it went. But so very many times these purchases would turn out to be mistakes. They would hang in my closet, never worn, and reproach me each time I looked at them. One day I was arguing with Carlo Jr. who wanted a new toy that he had seen in an advertisement. I told him that he couldn't just have anything he wanted because it amused him. I explained that he had plenty of toys and things to play with and that he had to learn to be content with what he already owned. The next time I felt the impulse to buy something, my words to Carlo came back to me. I realized I was behaving like a child, grabbing what caught my eye and that I needed a more realistic approach to shopping. I couldn't go on with the haphazard style of buying that left me, like a child with too many toys, with a closet full of clothes that weren't quite right.

My new approach begins with planning – which, as I have already said, is not my strong point. But what I do enjoy, before I even think about buying, is studying the fashion magazines. Even if I am not looking for something to buy, I love the photographs. Such fantasy and luxury . . . If I am traveling on a plane, I carefully pull out the photographs from the magazines when no one is looking and hide them to take home! Most of these items I would never think of buying, but they do have an effect on my final wardrobe decisions and they keep me up-to-date with the fashion world.

The main thing to avoid is going into a store with no idea of what you want. This can spell disaster and this is how you fill your closet with clothes you never wear. The magazines give you an idea of what is available and at what stores. Even if you spend half your shopping time at home just turning pages, I think this is time well spent.

Before you go to the store, you must also examine what you already have. It is simply wasteful to buy all new clothes every season; even if you have the money, and certainly not many people have, it means you haven't discovered what really is the best look for you. When you buy the right clothes, you should find that you can wear them for many seasons.

Look carefully through your wardrobe. Pick out the items that you have already worn and love. Think of how the new clothes you have seen in the magazines could be added to them. Think of what old pair of slacks could use a new blouse. Think about whether a new jacket would be just the thing to make an old dress look up-to-date. This can be the fun part of fashion. It is a challenge and it demands imagination.

Only after you have done all your fashion research are you ready to go into the store, and by then you should know exactly what you are looking for. You won't be wasting time wandering without direction. You will know what you want and won't be tempted to buy useless things.

When you shop, think in terms of outfits. If you are buying a new dress, be sure that you have the shoes, scarf and belt to go with it. Also, if you do see an impulse item that you can't resist, make certain that it will work as part of an outfit and not be an isolated, useless indulgence. This may mean that when you fall in love with a blouse, you must buy slacks to go with it. It may be more expensive but it is better than having a blouse you love and nothing to go with it.

Now that I have told you how practical I try to be about shopping, I must confess that there are times, often when I am with a friend, when I find myself buying some renegade item that catches my eye. But first I ask myself if I am going to wear it and if it will go with the other things I already have. If the answer is yes, I buy it, and I often find that these little purchases are wonderful additions to my wardrobe. And just occasionally I lose my heart to some bit of nonsense that is neither stylish nor elegant. I suppose it's like being attracted to a man you know is no good for you. But every now and again, it is fun to cast your fate to the wind. Sometimes the exceptions prove the rule.

The Elegant Uniform

Every woman has had that dark night of the fashion soul when she stands in front of her closet and cries to the heavens, "I haven't a thing to wear!" In my experience, it is women with closets bulging with clothes who most often face this dilemma. What makes the despair more powerful is that it is deepened by frustration and guilt. For it means that you have shopped much but not wisely. Moreover, I have a theory that each such despairing woman has an obsession for particular types of clothes. Everything she buys is much the same, so when the time comes, she can never decide what to wear. The trick is to discover what your own obsession is and then make it work for you.

My personal fashion obsession is comfort. Style, color and appropriateness all matter, but they take a backseat to total comfort. My goal is, once dressed, to become oblivious of my clothing. I hate a scarf that needs constant attention to keep it in place, or a waistband that binds, or a skirt that wraps itself around my legs. I have made my obsession work with my concept of "the elegant uniform." This for me is an outfit that looks good, is simple and comfortable, and can be worn at any time. Perhaps that dyed black ensemble I wore as a girl was the beginning of a lifelong habit!

The wonderful thing about an elegant uniform is that it eliminates the problem of wondering what to wear in the morning. I hate that because it is such a waste of time. With an elegant uniform I can dress quickly without a great deal of thought. Also I am sure that it will work because I choose my uniform carefully. When I feel good in my clothes, the whole day goes better.

If the fashion is good, one notices the person, not the clothes. That is a basic tenet of fashion and the elegant uniform surely adheres to it. But you must choose it with care: the word "elegant" is as important as "uniform."

My favorite elegant uniform begins with a pair of well-tailored black slacks. I sometimes try other neutral colors, but black goes with everything and looks good on me. When I find slacks that I really like, I buy two or three pairs. With them I vary the tops according to my mood and what my day holds. I might wear a bright silk blouse or a simple cotton shirt. It is easy to change the formality of the outfit by varying tops and accessories.

I love slacks. I think they are one of the great achievements of modern woman. This may sound frivolous, but think about it. Slacks free us to lead lives that are active and geared to achievement rather than lives confined by fussy clothes that imprison us as much as the home ever did. One thing to remember, however, is that wonderful as slacks are, their fit is crucial. They must be well cut and fit perfectly. Defects that could pass unnoticed in a skirt are emphasized in a pair of slacks.

In winter I add boots to my elegant uniform. I love boots and wear them everywhere: they are stylish and comfortable and they keep my feet warm and dry.

Bright scarves are accents that I use for variety. If I am going out, I might throw a beautiful print scarf around my neck. With boots and a black raincoat, I am prepared for anything.

If you want your own elegant uniform, first determine what your secret fashion obsession is. Is it for drama? Then buy some costume jewelry like dangling earrings or a glorious shawl. Is it for high fashion? Then buy an accessory, a belt, a scarf or even a jacket, that is dazzlingly stylish. Include these elements in your uniform, and you will always look elegant as well as being able to dress for the day in a flash.

Creative Accessories

Accessories are the items that can pull your wardrobe together and lift your look out of the ordinary. They give the finishing touch. Money can buy beautiful clothes, but it takes imagination and a sense of style to use accessories well.

You can make your wardrobe very elegant with only a few high-quality accessories. Even if you are on a budget, a good pair of boots, a beautiful scarf or fine gloves will add the look of luxury to a simple dress. Of course, you can use these items with other garments, and if you choose them well, they will last for a long time. Good accessories are a sound fashion investment.

Finally, accessories will add your own distinctive touch to a wardrobe. Many women may own the same dress, but it is the way they complete their look that will give them distinction. With accessories you can express a mood or create a unique impression; they give you an opportunity to use creativity and imagination.

Perfume, the Intimate Accessory

Perfume, like silk, wine and fresh flowers, to me is one of the necessary luxuries of life. A particular joy of perfume is that it has such a powerful effect on your mood, lending confidence and glamor, romance and elegance at a touch.

Did you know that our memory for smells is more accurate and

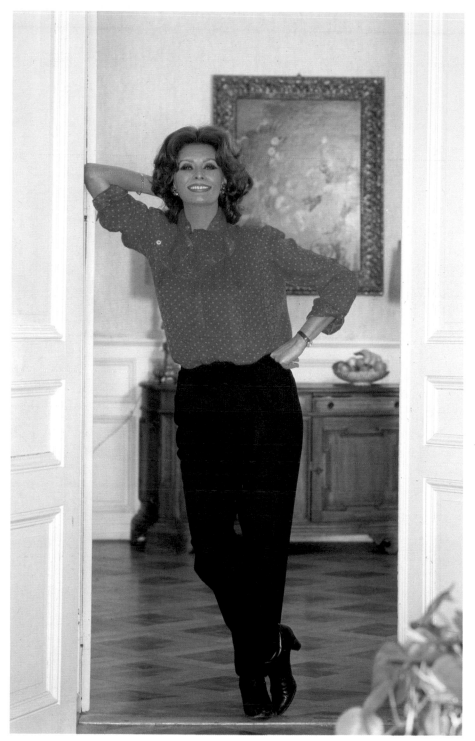

My own special 'elegant uniform' – well-cut black slacks,
dramatized here by a bright red shirt.

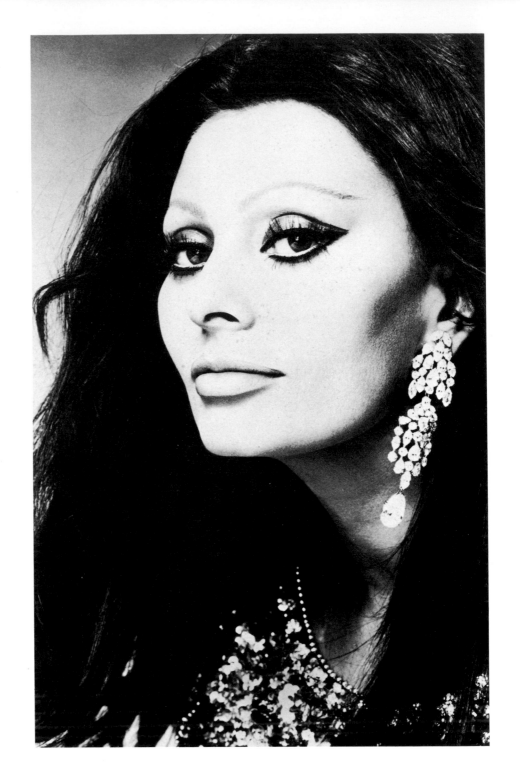

One of my most popular fan pictures, taken in the mid-seventies.

long-lasting than it is for any of the other senses? We have all had the experience of being transported back to our childhood by a smell that we remember so clearly and distinctly that we are amazed. For me, the smell of the sea has this effect. Also the odor of a barn always pleases me, perhaps because it takes me back to the barns of my childhood, where my mother found milk for me during the war. Even now when I smell this aroma, I feel warm and cozy and cared for.

Because perfume is such a direct route to the unconscious, it can become a personal signature and remembrance for our loved ones, carrying with its scent many memories and associations.

Choose a perfume carefully and don't rush the process. Scent is like a fine wine that needs to breathe before it reaches perfection. It takes about thirty minutes to develop fully on the skin. You can't go into a store, sniff a few scents and then choose. The best way is to try a single scent, wear it for a few hours, then decide how you feel about it. The next day, try another. Eventually you will find one that suits you.

As to the use of perfume, remember that "love and perfume you must not hoard." It can be one of the most emotionally appealing of all accessories. Use if freely. And since it can be very expensive, you should look after it. Sunlight affects it and so do extremes of heat and cold. Also, once the bottle is opened, oxygen will begin to change the scent. Perfume is supposed to have a life of three years, but I think it is wise to buy only enough for one year at a time. That way you are sure that it will last in good condition.

Jewelry

When I first began to achieve some success in my career, I loved buying and wearing jewels. To me they were a status symbol. They made me believe that I was really living the dreams I had had for so long. They represented conquest and achievement.

But then I had terrible trouble because of my jewelry. I was robbed twice, and since those experiences I no longer wear real gems. Expensive stones are not possessions but threats: you have to insure them and be careful how you wear them in public and always worry about them. I think life is difficult enough these days and I see no reason to make it more so for the sake of fancy stones and metal. So I seldom wear real jewels, except on very special occasions when I will be in the public eye, or in some connection with my work. But the jewels are borrowed. I wear them for one night and in the morning, back they go where someone else can worry about them.

One of the other troubles with expensive jewelry is that you run the danger of people noticing the gems rather than you. I have often heard a woman say to another at a party, "Goodness, did you see the necklace she is

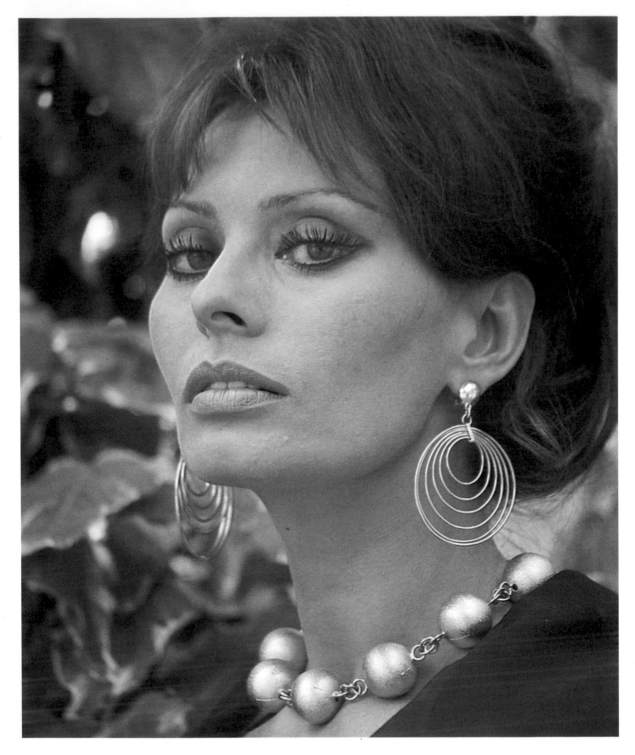

I think it is more interesting to combine different types of jewelry.

wearing?" This means that the adornment has become more important than the woman. I don't like the idea of wearing jewelry so that it is noticed for its price, nor do I like jewels to detract from me and the way I look. A necklace or an earring should add to your glamor but not because of its cost; after all, it is an ornament, nothing more.

Still, I do like to wear jewelry because it completes a look and flatters your face. So I wear fake gems. Today we are lucky because some costume jewelry is so beautifully made that you really can't distinguish it from the real thing. Of course, the best imitation pieces are not cheap, but they are not nearly as expensive as the real ones, and you don't have to worry when you wear them.

One mistake to avoid when wearing jewelry is having too many matching pieces at the same time. A bracelet and a necklace and earrings and rings that all go together often look really boring. Vary your combinations to give more visual interest. Remember as well to limit the number of items you wear. Some women fall into the trap of wearing too much jewelry and then it detracts from their appearance rather than enhancing it.

Hats

I must have a weakness for hats – I have owned so many in my life! I really enjoy them because they are fun and also dramatic; they can give you a very elegant or even whimsical look. When a woman wears a hat she is memorable. And nothing puts the finishing touch on an outfit like a hat. A hat will also protect your hair from weather and the sun, and on those days when you don't have much time to devote to your hair, a hat can be an elegant disguise.

I was lucky to meet a man in Paris who is truly an artist with hats. Jean Barthet takes straw or felt or paper and before your eyes, like a sculptor he shapes something that eventually becomes a beautiful, charming hat that is just right for you. We became great friends, and whenever I need a hat I go to him. He invented a style called a "casquette" just for me. It has a narrow brim in the front and a round top. I have casquettes in a few different sorts of fur, and I have been wearing them for twenty years. Barthet's genius is that every hat he makes is sure to flatter the person who wears it. Of course, he does not make a lot of money because like an artist he does all the work himself by hand. He did, however, make a line of hats for fashionable American stores like Bloomingdale's, and if you are lucky you may find one of them.

Shopping for hats in a department store that has a good selection is great fun if you go with a friend, because you can go from hat to hat, and try on whatever is available without having to wait for a dressing room. There are

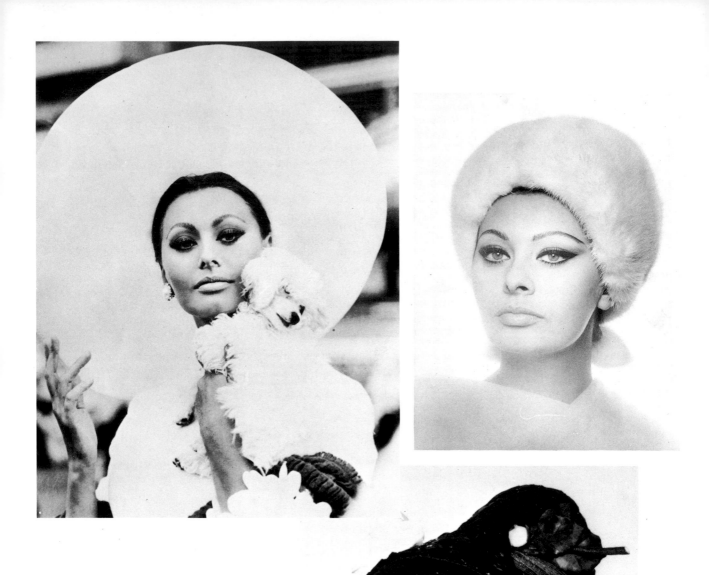

I love hats, in every shape and form.

_____

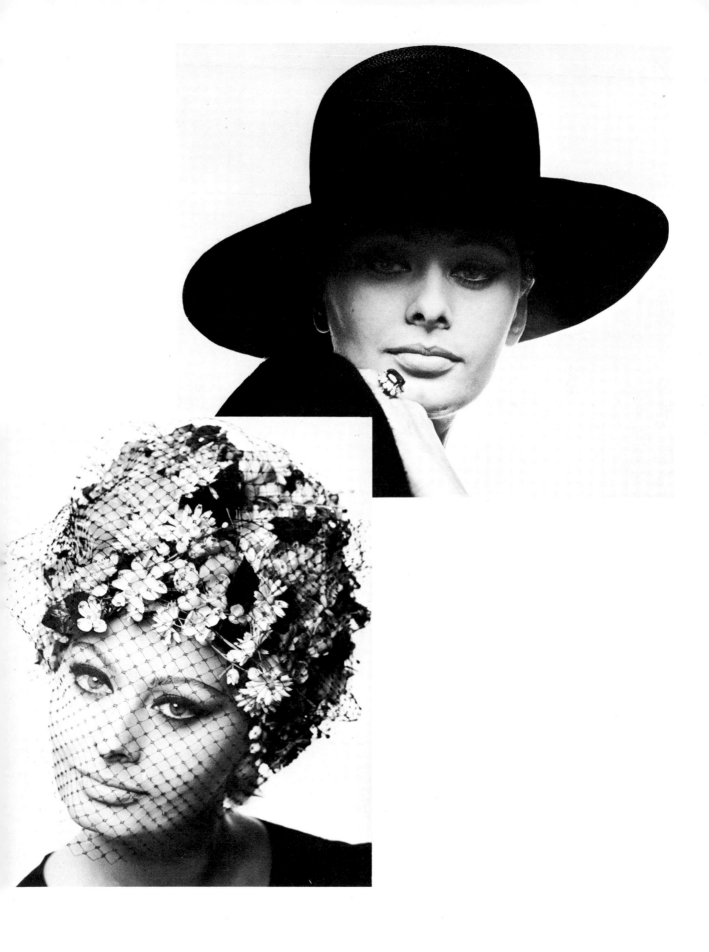

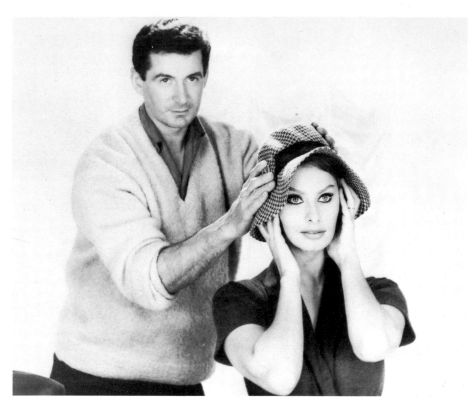

With my friend Jean Barthet, a true genius in the art of hat-making, in Paris in the sixties.

---

some styles like berets that I think almost everyone can wear. But if you want to buy a more unusual shape you must choose carefully. Be sure the brim and the crown are the right size for your face and hairstyle. Some faces are dwarfed by a large brim, and some heads look too magnified in a large crown. Check too that the proportion of the hat works with your body. Sometimes a large hat on a very short woman can be completely overpowering, and on a tall woman a tiny hat may simply disappear. Try on the hat in front of a full-length mirror so you are sure that it is in proportion with your size.

You also need to be careful that the mood of your hat matches the mood of your face. I have seen women with very sad faces wearing very funny hats, and it is incongruous. You need the right attitude for your hat, or it won't work for you.

Also be sure when you buy a hat that it goes with your outfit. You should not wear an extravagantly fussy creation with a suit or a very informal cap with an elegant outfit.

One type of summer hat that I think is wonderful and goes with most warm-weather fashions is a natural straw hat. It always looks fresh and unpretentious and pretty; with some flowers or a simple colored ribbon on the brim, it can make you feel like a girl in springtime.

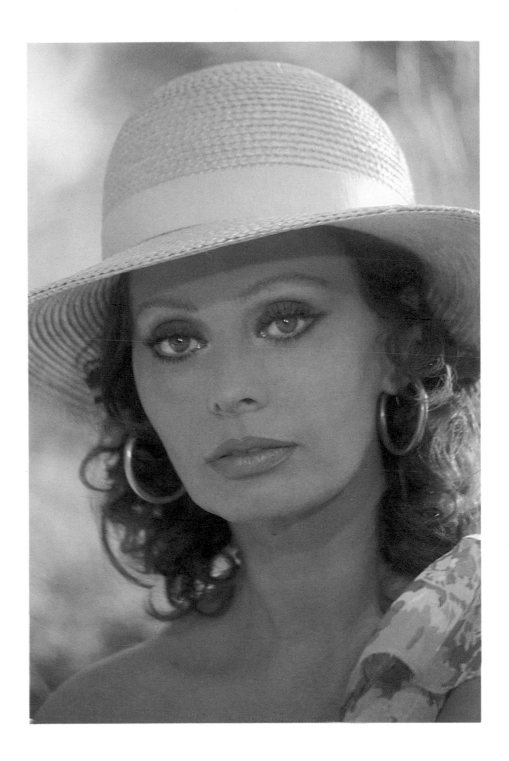

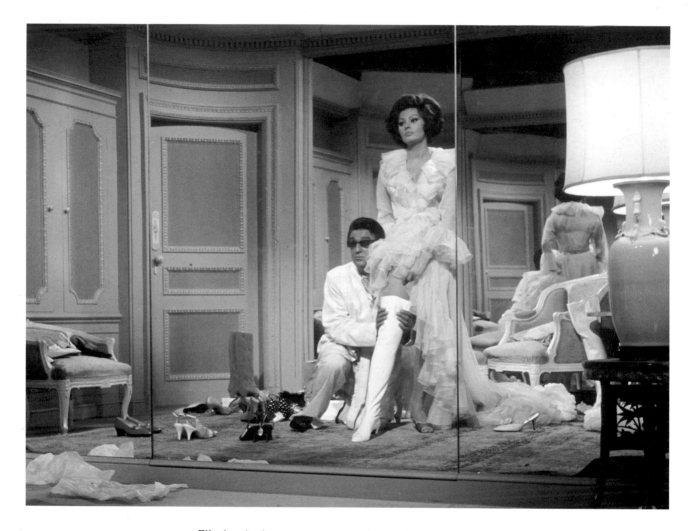

Filming Arabesque *gave me plenty of scope for indulging my passion for shoes.*

Shoes

If I have an extravagant streak in my soul, most of it is expressed in my lust for shoes. Perhaps unconsciously I think of shoes as a kind of sculpture, and indeed they are – some are extraordinary works of art with their cantilevered platforms, delicate straps, and expressive heels and toes. I find them irresistible and add some to my collection regularly. Perhaps one day I will open a shoe museum to encourage the appreciation of this neglected art. Unfortunately, this same quality of art and sculpture is what makes many shoes more appropriate to a museum than a foot.

For many women, myself included, buying a pair of shoes is like a brief, sad love affair – the desire, the satisfaction, the disillusionment, the pain, all condensed into one afternoon. There is a more sinister aspect to uncomfortable shoes which I once heard a cynic express this way: "Yes, they are beautiful, those shoes, but notice how cruel. The young girl starts out in shoes like delicate canoes but ends her life in ocean liners." This is a sad fact of life if you regularly sacrifice comfort for fashion where your feet are concerned. Eventually your poor feet will be tormented into corns and callouses and bunions, and then you will be forced to wear ocean liners in order to walk. These words stuck with me, and even though I have dozens of pairs of beautiful shoes, I wear the same ones all the time – the few pairs that are really comfortable and fit well.

When filming, I am sometimes forced to wear very high heels or uncomfortable shoes for long periods of time, and it is amazing how tired they make you feel and how soon your legs and back begin to ache. Recently in New York I was delighted to see young women walking around the city in comfortable sneakers, carrying more formal shoes in their bags. This isn't the most elegant look, but to me these running shoes are an emblem of freedom. Walking is my favorite exercise and it is a kind of slavery for women to be forced to hobble in high heels.

My other major piece of advice for you concerning shoes is to avoid white. When a woman wears white shoes they are the only things you see. I watched myself once in an early film wearing white pumps and my feet looked like Minnie Mouse's – I don't have big feet but those white shoes somehow managed to fill the screen!

If you have very nice legs, almost any type of shoe will look pretty on you, but if you have a problem with your legs as to shape or size, you will have to choose more carefully. For example, heavy legs or thick ankles are emphasized by ankle straps. If you have either of these, you should look for shoes that are cut low in the front, if possible nearly to the top of the toes, for this will give the illusion of length to the leg.

Boots are flattering on any woman and can disguise a multitude of sins. I am a bit like an American cowboy in my devotion to boots. I wear them all the time in the winter because they are so comfortable, and they look equally polished and chic with slacks or with a skirt. Shop carefully until you find boots with a good heel height for you and a versatile look – one that can go with both casual and more dressy clothes. Be very fussy when you buy boots and get the best quality you can afford. If you treat them well with polish, and waterproof them when they need it, your boots will last a long time.

I must tell you that for my feet and probably yours, the best shoe is none at all. I go barefoot whenever I can because it is such a fine way to relax the feet and legs. Walking in the sand at the beach will please your feet better than the most expensive shoes, and it provides the best possible exercise for your feet and legs, firming your muscles as it removes rough skin. It is a good idea to wear flat shoes or slippers whenever you can, especially if you must wear high heels for work. By varying the height of your heels you use different muscles in your legs, thus keeping them more flexible and shapely. And finally, if you want the happiest feet in the world, do as I have done and teach your children or loved one to massage your feet.

Scarves

Scarves are one of the most versatile accessories we have today. You can wear a scarf as a necklace, a hat, a belt, a shawl, a skirt or even a dress. Every woman, no matter what her personal style, can extend her wardrobe by using scarves.

I have a good collection of scarves and, unlike my shoes, this collection is in constant use. Recently I bought some scarves from Dior, Saint Laurent and Valentino that are among the most beautiful I have ever seen – they are like paintings, with luminous colors and artistic designs. When I wear my black raincoat with one of these scarves, I feel like a million dollars, even if I am only going to the post office.

Scarves are wonderful as color accents and this is how I usually use them. As I have said, I love to dress in black but total blackness can sometimes be too severe. So I add a brilliant scarf, usually at the neck, and the black moves into another dimension. In the same vein, you will find that colors you love but aren't flattering, will work for you in a scarf. So a pretty green or saffron color that in a blouse might dull your skin will look fine when accenting a print scarf.

There is another quality about scarves that is as valuable as their versatility and their color. Flung around the neck, blowing in a breeze, drifting on the night air, scarves have a romance about them. I suppose it is partly due to the movement they give to clothes as they echo the motion of our bodies and of the air: they float and drift with a sensuousness that can be very erotic. Scarves are useful props for a girl with romance on her mind. I too always feel a thrill of romance and adventure when silk floats around my collar, and this is one of the secret pleasures of scarves.

Glasses

Have you ever heard the rhyme "Men don't make passes at girls who wear glasses"? Don't believe it for a minute! On the contrary, I think many men secretly cherish the fantasy of a woman taking off her glasses and unpinning

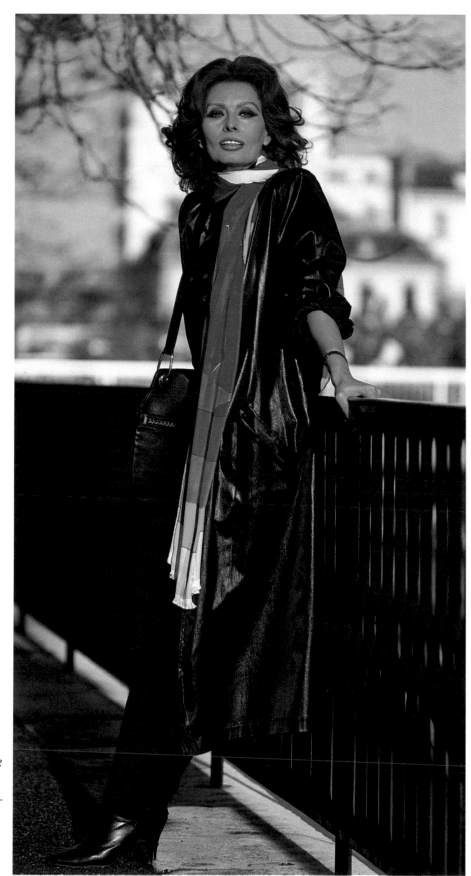

I love the dramatic impact of a brightly colored scarf with a dark outfit.

her hair and becoming a tigress. Can you imagine this scene played out with contact lenses?

I wear glasses and consider them a fashion accessory. In fact, I have my own line of eyeframes with Zyloware that I have chosen personally because I think women deserve frames that are pretty and flattering. After all, glasses are like a hairstyle or jewelry – something that people notice about you right away. Because of this, you should choose them with all the care you devote to other accessories, and think about how they will affect your overall appearance rather than just your eyes or your face. Don't be shy about taking your time and asking the advice of friends. Sometimes it can be difficult to judge yourself how the frames work with your face and hair.

Try to select a frame that is in proportion to your face. If you have wide-set eyes, a larger frame will be more flattering. If your eyes are close-set, choose a smaller frame. Apart from this, I think you simply have to keep trying on frames until you find a shape that flatters your face.

There is a wide range of choice today in the color of frames. Naturally you will want to pick a shade that complements the main colors in your wardrobe. For example, if you wear mainly blues and grays, then blue or even burgundy-tinted frames will look good. If you choose your wardrobe from a brown or neutral palette, you might choose brown or beige frames. Of course, neutral-colored frames are always safe and versatile.

Don't forget to coordinate the color of the frame with your hair color. If you have light hair – gray or blond – you will probably find that light-colored frames will be best, while a dark-haired woman will look better in dark frames that balance the color of her hair.

You might want to try some tinted lenses to see if they suit you: they can be very sophisticated and also flattering to your face. But remember that the color of the lenses too should harmonize with your wardrobe, so if you wear a great variety of colors and are buying only one pair of eyeglasses, you may find that tinted lenses clash with much of what you wear.

If you can afford them, it is nice to have a special pair of eyeglasses for evening wear. There are some elegant metal frames with a gold or silver finish which look wonderful with gold or silver jewelry, while transparent or opaline frames complement pearls very well.

A final practical note for those of us who wear eyeglasses: nothing spoils a polished look more quickly than lenses that look as if they have just survived a dust storm. It makes a very bad impression – like arriving at the Ritz in a jalopy. You may be able to see the rest of the world through dirty lenses, but it won't be able to see you. So carry a packet of paper optical tissues in your purse and make a habit of cleaning your lenses regularly.

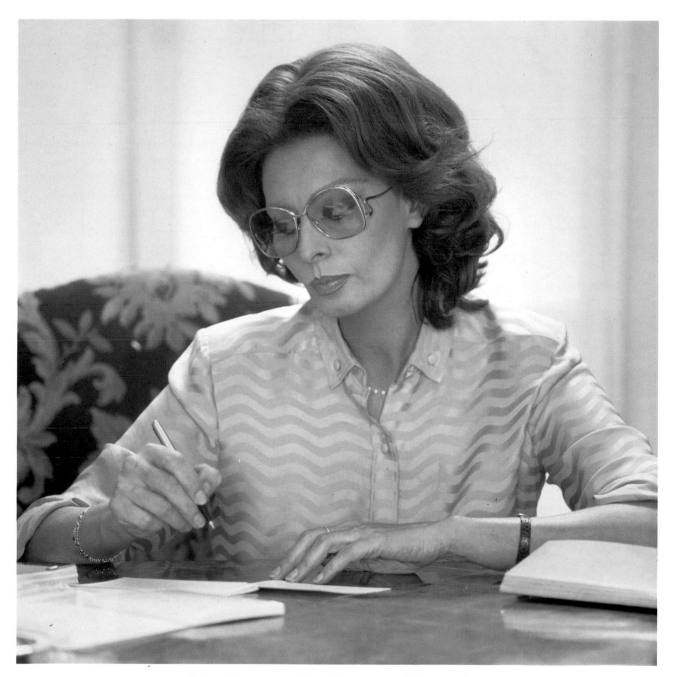

Colored frames and tinted lenses should harmonize with the clothes you wear, as well as flattering your complexion.

A HEALTHY DIET

When Peter Sellers began his career in films, he was overweight. In his first important film, *The Mouse That Roared,* he was positively plump. I was to star with him in his next film, *The Millionairess,* and as I had never seen him act, the producers brought a copy of *The Mouse* to me in Switzerland. I loved the film and was crazy about Peter's acting and very pleased that we would be working together. But the producers were worried about his weight. He had promised them he would lose half his total weight by the time we started filming. This seemed impossible to me but, sure enough, when I met him just before we began the picture, he was a new man. It made a big difference to his career: at last, his comic genius was able to shine through. I know that it wasn't easy for him to lose weight, but because he was highly motivated he managed to do so.

People who have a serious problem with weight, who need to lose a great deal, sometimes need a special, dramatic event to push them to action. Sometimes professional help is called for. If you are one of these people, I urge you to get the necessary help. Find a doctor or a nutritionist who will instruct you and inspire you and help you find the moral courage you will need. Remember that serious obesity is not a beauty problem; it is a medical problem. If you are more than fifteen or twenty pounds overweight, you are damaging your health even more than your appearance.

My weight has never been a problem for me. I have gained a few pounds for a time and then lost them again. When George Cukor directed me in *Heller in Pink Tights,* he wanted me to lose some weight to conform to a certain look he had in mind. I lost the weight without trouble. In fact, in that film I was thinner than ever before or since in my life. I am amused to see the photographs of me in costume with what looks like a fifteen-inch waist. To be honest, I should tell you that in certain costumes, even though I was very slim, I had to wear one of those corsets that are laced up until you almost can't breathe.

Just because I have never had a weight problem, it doesn't mean that I never give a thought to food. After all, what you eat affects the way you look, and when you are a film actress, the way you look is magnified many times on the screen. Diet is important not only to your figure, but also to your good health, your complexion, even your state of mind.

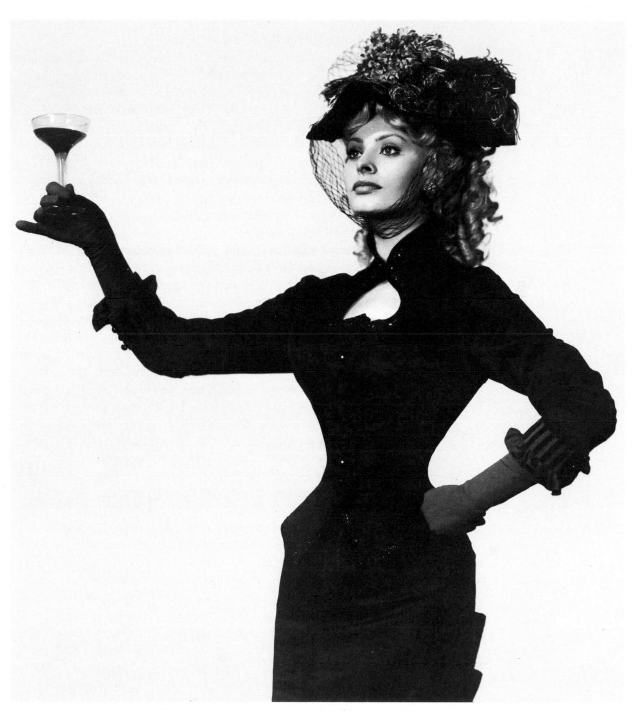

Showing off my wasp waist in Heller in Pink Tights.

The Tyranny of the Endless Diet

Women today are obsessed by extra weight, and many of them have made their lives very difficult by starving themselves into nervous, weak creatures who are chronically depressed because they believe they are a few pounds overweight. I have seen women at dinner parties who are so thin that their shoulders could be weapons and they eat nothing because they are "watching their calories." I have known women who have wasted years of their lives by believing that they are too fat to be glamorous. They dread shopping for clothes, they hate to dress up for an occasion, they complain about the smallest bulge on their waistlines or thighs as if it were a failure of the greatest magnitude. In Italy we call these women *attaccapanni,* which means coathanger, because that is what they resemble.

Before I begin to say anything specific about diet and exercise, I want to tell you that if you are constantly worried about your figure and always afraid to eat, the problem lies not in your body but in your mind. The first thing you need to do is realize that life is more than the absence of fat. If the shape of your body is a serious worry to you, then you should do something about it, but you must recognize what is a problem and what is not. A little extra weight is nothing. Put it out of your mind. Follow my simple advice about nutrition and exercise and you will probably find that you lose some pounds as if by accident. But don't postpone living until you reach the perfect size. Don't think that when you lose a few pounds you will be happy, or when you can fit into a smaller size, life will begin for you. I can't emphasize strongly enough that this is a tragic attitude. A feeling of inferiority about what you consider to be excess weight will do you far more damage than the weight itself.

Women have made so many advances in society today and are so free, but one thing that still seems to chain them is a morbid fear of a round tummy or a dimpled thigh. I remember meeting Ella Fitzgerald and being enormously impressed by her energy and her pride. She is a big woman with a powerful physique, but the fact that her figure does not conform to a fashion model's standards of what is correct does not give her a moment's pause. She looks wonderful in colorful caftans and sweeping dresses, and her strong body serves only to make her more attractive. She doesn't hold herself back because she is convinced that she must lose a few pounds; she is leading a full and successful life on her own terms. I urge you to do the same.

Nutrition

Food is one of the few weapons we have readily at hand in our fight to maintain good health. Naturally you don't walk barefoot in the snow and you don't go without sleep for three days. Yet the same people who care in every other way for their bodies think that if their hunger is satisfied and their clothes fit, their diet is good. They will eat anything they feel like eating and worry only if they start to gain weight. They would probably be shocked by someone who poured any old liquid into the gas tank of a car and still expected it to work, yet that is really what they are doing with their bodies.

It is surprising that most of us know so little about a subject that has such a big effect on our lives. I suppose this is because we are lucky to live in a time when for many people food is in good supply. Indeed, it is probably because food is so plentiful that we are inclined to overeat and eat indiscriminately. But the human body depends on good nutrition to operate properly. I think that many of the nervous symptoms we experience today – headaches, insomnia, fatigue, allergies and so on – are the signs of a body that is slightly out of order because it is not getting the proper fuel. Learning something about nutrition is sensible not only for the sake of our figures but also for our health.

I took my first real interest in nutrition after my boys were born because here were two creatures who depended on me entirely for their food. I had to know what would be the best foods for them. So I learned about the different food groups and about fats and carbohydrates and proteins. I advise every woman to learn these things, not only for her children but for herself. Once you know the basics of what you should be eating every day you will choose your food more wisely, and you will also understand why it is such a mistake to fill yourself with foods that do you no good and only add weight and probably make you sick.

I don't aim to go into great detail on nutrition here because there are already a whole host of books on the subject. But I have some basic recommendations for you to keep in mind when you shop and cook and sit down to eat.

> Try to eat three balanced meals every day. Having just coffee is not a good way to begin the day, and I try, even though I have little appetite in the morning, to eat some fruit or bread to give my body a start on the day's work. Lunch for me is often the big meal of the day, when I will have pasta, a bit of meat or fish, perhaps a salad and coffee. The evening meal is a light version of lunch with the addition of wine. Each meal should be eaten at leisure, and pleasure should play a big role. I look forward especially to dinner because the boys are back from school and we share the day's news.

> I believe that it is a mistake to skip meals because you are dieting or to sit at a meal and only sip water or juice. You will just

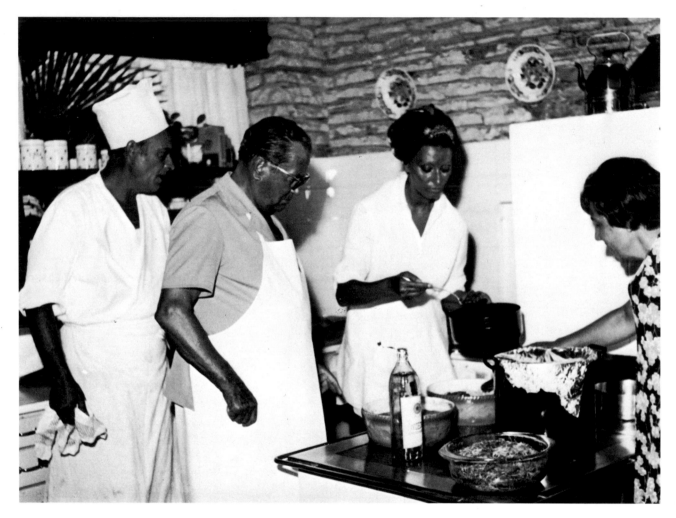

I love any excuse to learn about cooking. Here I am with the late President Tito of Yugoslavia in his kitchen on the island of Brioni, in the Adriatic. I taught him the secret of a good meat sauce, and he introduced me to the mysteries of moussaka.

be hungry later and will be tempted to overeat. Even if that isn't the case, you can't expect your body to function at its best without food. If you are trying to control your weight, do what I do: eat three meals a day but take small portions.

I was interested to read recently of an experiment carried out to learn when and how the body uses food. In this experiment people in three groups ate all the same foods at different times of day: one group ate only in the morning, one at noon and the third in the evening. The morning group lost weight, the noon group stayed the same and the evening group gained weight. It seems that the earlier you eat, the better use the body makes of that food. This would argue for a good breakfast and a small dinner. Ironically, that is just the reverse of the way most people eat.

Do not snack. Here is a rule that, in my experience, is most often broken in America, but the problem unfortunately is beginning to circle the globe. Eating snacks between meals is the enemy of good nutrition. For one thing, you are never really hungry because you are always nibbling, but although you have little appetite for meals, you still eat them out of habit or because they are a social event.

Not only does eating continual snacks add weight, it also makes you tired. This is because after you eat a meal your body is preoccupied with the task of digestion: the blood rushes to your digestive tract where it is needed to digest the food, which is why you feel tired after a meal. If you eat all the time, you will find that you always feel a little tired because your body is always busy digesting.

Of course, there is nothing wrong with having a small piece of fruit or some juice during the day. It is the potato chips (which I love, by the way, but avoid because they are so fattening and so hard to stop eating), and the candy and all the other salty, fattening snacks that we usually eat out of boredom or habit rather than because we are hungry – these are the snacks that should be avoided.

Try to avoid processed foods. It is wonderful to have so much choice all during the year of those foods that used to be seasonal only – and it is handy to be able to prepare a meal in an instant after a busy day. But still I think we shouldn't allow convenience to rob us of the pleasure of working with fresh foods whenever possible. I feel this way because I enjoy cooking and I take a sensuous pleasure in working with my hands with fresh foods instead of using a can opener. But even if you don't enjoy cooking, you should favor fresh foods because they are so much better for you. They contain more of the vitamins and minerals your body needs to convert food into energy, and in my opinion, they certainly taste better than processed foods.

Drink plenty of liquids during the day. Did you know that very

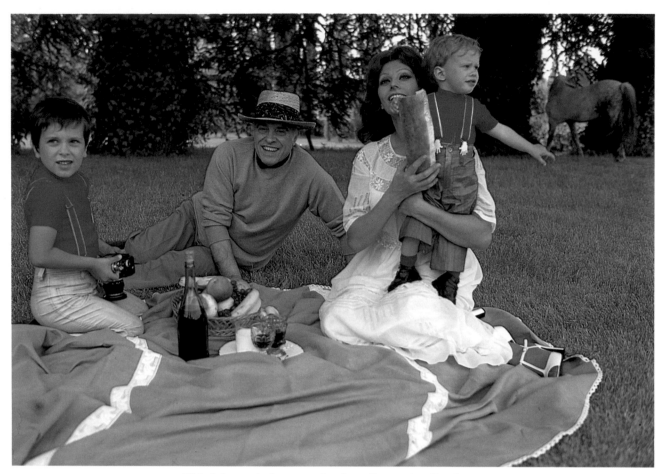

*This informal photograph of us all on a family picnic was taken
in the garden at Marino in 1975.*

often when you think you are hungry, you are really thirsty? Drinking not only works to satisfy you, it is also crucial in cleansing your body of impurities.

Sometimes women have a problem with fluid retention. Their eyes are puffy in the morning and their ankles swell. If you suffer in this way, do not cut down on water, for this only makes things worse by reducing the body's ability to flush wastes.

Eat less red meat and more fish and chicken. White meats and fish contain less fat and every bit as much protein as red meat. In any event, most people eat far more protein than they need and would do well to cut down on their protein intake. But the big problem with red meat is the fat; even if you cut off all visible fat, the best and most juicy steak is marbled throughout with fat, which will add unneeded calories to your diet and cholesterol to your circulatory system.

Finally, some good news: eat more pasta! At last, I have support from scientists as well as gourmets when I urge pasta upon you. So many times people have asked, while covertly gazing at my hips or waistline, how I keep my figure with all that pasta. Now the tagalong scientists have confirmed what Italian mamas have known for generations – pasta is good for you. Indeed, Italians are lucky to live with a culinary heritage that relies on pasta because it is a complex carbohydrate and a very efficient and healthy fuel for the body. Complex carbohydrates are also found in beans, rice and vegetables. Eating carbohydrates will keep you from getting hungry by preventing your blood-sugar level from dropping. Scientists have found that it is easiest to lose weight on a diet rich in complex carbohydrates for that very reason: the carbohydrates will satisfy your hunger and give you energy because they are being burned efficiently by your body.

The best pasta for good nutrition is whole-wheat pasta – we call it black pasta in Italy. Of course, you can't expect to add rich cream sauces and still enjoy its good effects. Serve the pasta with a sauce made of tomatoes and unrefined olive oil, with perhaps some shredded carrots added for natural sweetness.

Once when I was making one of my pasta sauces, my cook Lydia, who is pleasantly plump, told me that you can gain weight just from breathing the kitchen aromas. At first, I thought this was Lydia's excuse for not being slim, but gradually I realized it was her way of getting me out of the kitchen!

THE VALUE OF EXERCISE

*R*egular exercise is absolutely essential to a healthy body, and I think it is as important for your spirits as for your body. But the fact is, I am not an athletic woman. The idea of doing rounds of calisthenics bores me. When I came to Los Angeles a few years ago and saw everyone running down the street, I thought the long-awaited earthquake had finally arrived. I wondered why everyone was leaving their children behind in their rush to flee the city. Then I learned that they were running for exercise and fun!

I have never jogged and I never will. It is not a good exercise for me because it jolts my body too much. I cannot believe all that pounding is good for you. A doctor in New York told me that he is beginning to come across foot, knee and ankle problems in people who jog, and he believes that as joggers get older, these problems will get worse. I also think that running in cities, in which your lungs are asked to filter out all that polluted air, cannot be good for your health.

To me, exercise is not a matter of fashion. Though it is really a small part of my life in terms of hours, I take exercise very seriously and I would never just adopt the latest popular routine unless I were positive that it was good for my body.

As you can guess, I am not going to tell you that you must start lifting weights or run around the city or hang upside down from your ceiling. I am going to tell you what I – a woman who prefers poker to parachuting and Scrabble to skiing – do to keep my body in shape.

The Argument for Exercise

We all know that we should exercise, but the reasons for doing so are often vague. "It will make you feel better," perhaps. Yes, but so will a nap or a warm bath. I have always exercised because it keeps my body firm, but only recently have I learned some of the really excellent reasons for exercising.

> Contrary to what most women think, exercise will decrease your appetite and help you burn more calories even hours after you have stopped. To me this is almost a miracle. I have always noticed that after I exercise, I am not hungry, but just imagine –

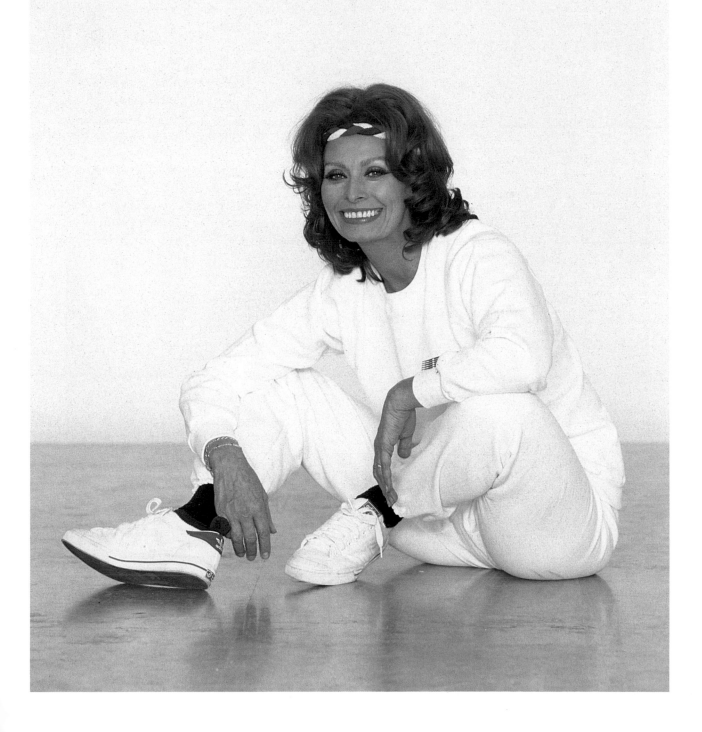

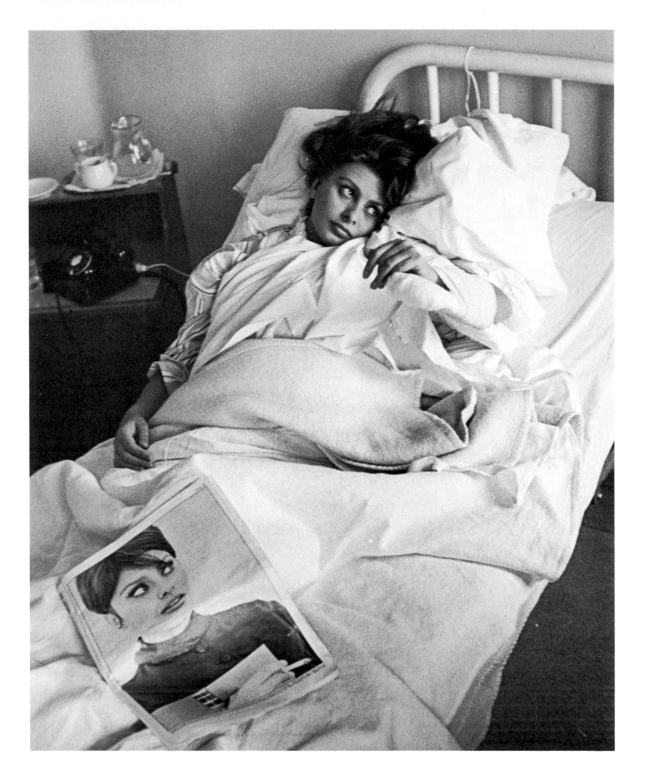

The result of my fall on the last day of shooting El Cid.

not only does your appetite decrease, your body continues to burn calories more rapidly than ever for hours afterward. It is as if you started a fire that continues to burn long after the kindling has gone out. This means that your body's increased metabolism is working to keep you trim and firm far beyond your actual exercise time. What a wonderful dividend that is.

Exercise reduces stress, anxiety and related nervous problems as well as relieving depression. It has been proven that exercise that raises your heatbeat for at least fifteen minutes causes your brain to release a substance that gives a boost to the brain's pleasure centers. Naturally this makes you feel good. Even if you are not feeling depressed, you will find that exercise will make you more cheerful. My own theory is that the very discipline of exercising also gives a sense of self-control and achievement that is exhilarating.

There have been times in my life, usually in the midst of filming, when I haven't been able to fit in my usual amount of walking, my favorite exercise. I realize how much I miss it when I am deprived for a few days. When we were filming *El Cid*, we were working very hard at the end and I couldn't find time to go on the long daily walk that I enjoyed. The lack of exercise, combined with the pressure of finishing the film, made me unusually tense, and on the final day of shooting, I fell down a flight of stairs. Being tense makes anyone clumsy and I certainly paid for my lack of exercise.

Exercise helps you sleep. This is obvious, but sometimes we forget. Exercise will tire your muscles and relax you so that you go to sleep more quickly and sleep more soundly. Remember how you used to fall into bed as a child, exhausted from the day's play? You can experience that same wonderful fatigue by exercising regularly.

Exercise increases the strength of your bones. This was interesting news to me. We all know that as we age, our bones become brittle. This can be a serious problem for elderly women if they fall and break a hip or leg. But when you exercise, you increase the calcium in the bones. They become stronger and better able to withstand the stresses and jolts of everyday life.

Exercise makes you more graceful. When you exercise you walk as if you own the street – with pride and fluidity.

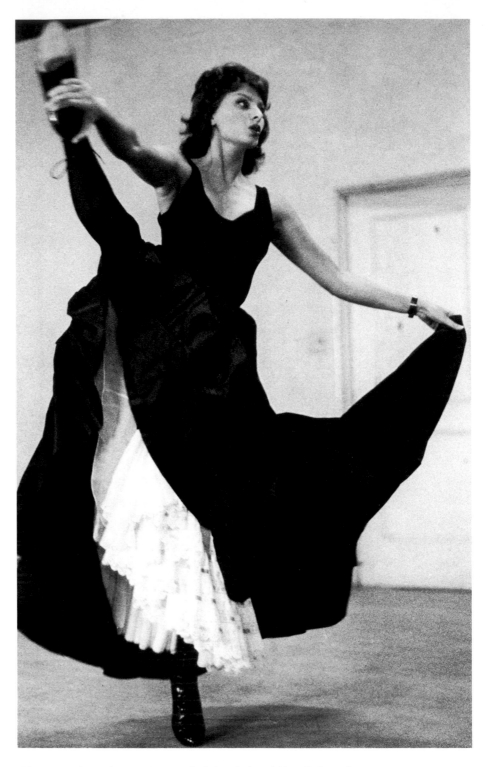

My career has always demanded that I should be fit: here I am doing a high kick in Heller in Pink Tights.

My Exercise Program

My approach to exercise is very simple and practical because it has to be. Being an actress is like being a mother – your time is not your own. I am an actress and a mother, so it is doubly difficult for me to have a rigid exercise routine. I could not, for example, depend on any kind of equipment because if I made a film in the desert, as I have done, or had to spend weeks going from hotel room to hotel room, as I have also done, I would then lack the means to keep up with my exercise routine.

There are three parts to my exercise program: stretching, walking and trouble spots. The stretching keeps me limber and graceful, the walking gets my blood circulating – and the trouble spots are a collection of exercises that I use for special areas that need toning or strengthening.

Stretching

You have probably seen a cat or a dog in the morning when it gets up. The first thing it does is take a luxurious stretch that works nearly every muscle in its body. We have two dogs, and it amazes me to see them rest their chests on the floor, bottoms to the sky, while they stretch out their front legs, chests and backs. Then they stretch out their hindlegs, dragging them along the floor. Again they stretch their backs and finally their necks and heads as they point their noses to the sky, holding the pose briefly. It is really quite a production – like a morning at the Kirov ballet.

I think the animals have a lesson for us. I follow their lead in almost every movement except the final shake, which I have never been able to master! Every morning as soon as I get up, I do a brief but I believe very effective routine of simple stretches. Before I learned about the other benefits of exercising, I knew that these stretches were good for me. They get my blood circulating in the morning. They bring a nice rush of color to my face. But the most important thing is that they keep me supple. Some mornings I wake up with a little ache or stiffness, but by the time I have finished with my stretches, I am limber and relaxed.

I also make a point of breathing deeply when I do my stretches. A friend who practices Chinese medicine in Rome told me that we regularly use only a tiny percentage of our lungs when we do our usual shallow breathing. He said that deep, regular breathing brings oxygen to all of the lungs, purifies the blood and give us great energy and tranquility. Since having that conversation with him, I have made a point of working on my breathing and I think it really makes a difference. When doing these stretches, try to fill your lungs with as much air as you can. Let your stomach expand as you inhale – don't try to pull it in until you exhale. When you exhale, push out every bit of stale air.

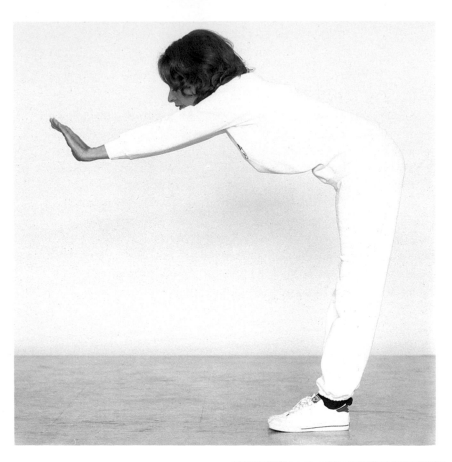

TOE TOUCH   Bend over from the waist, keeping your knees straight. Let your arms and your head hang down, fingers toward the floor. You will feel your back and leg muscles stretching. The point is not to force yourself to touch your toes, but to let gravity do the work for you and gently stretch your muscles. Don't bounce or you will find that the muscles you want to stretch become tight. I do this stretch two of three times.

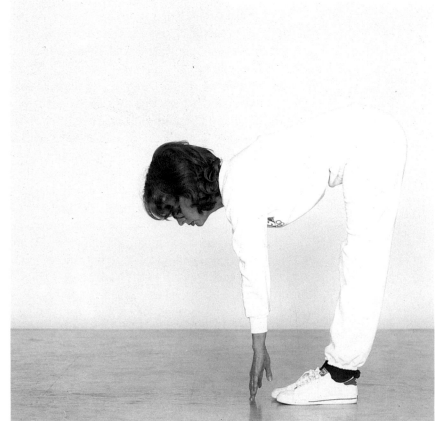

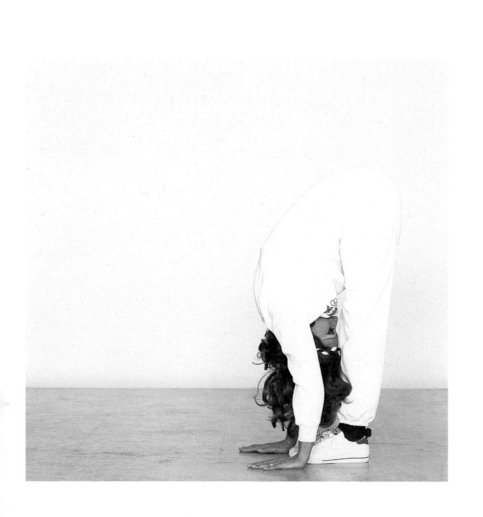

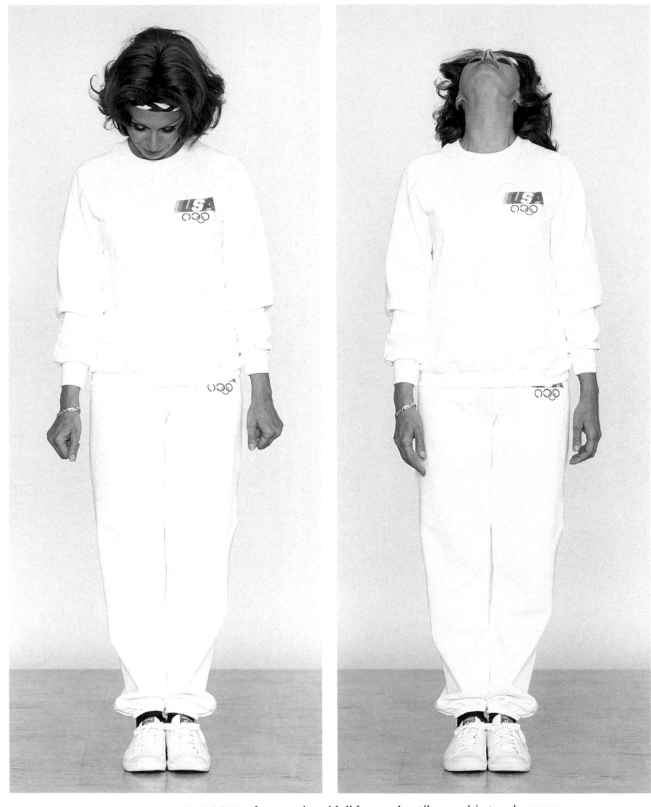

HEAD ROLL   Let your head fall forward until your chin touches your chest. Then let it fall backward so you are looking at the ceiling.

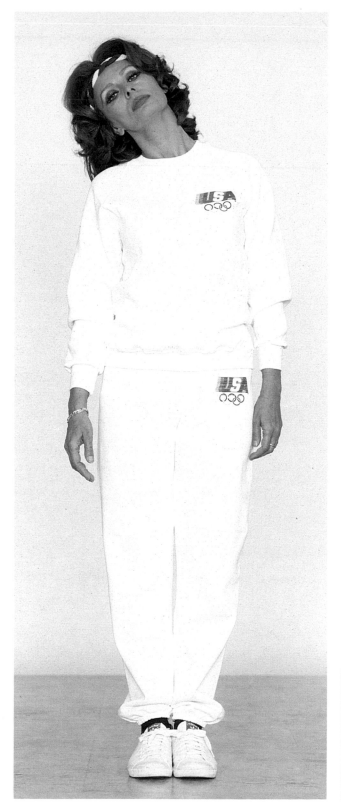
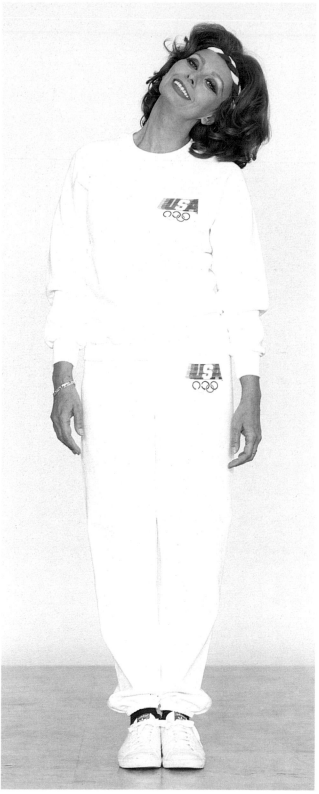

Then, holding your shoulders down, let your head fall from side to side. In each movement, feel the muscles in the neck stretch.

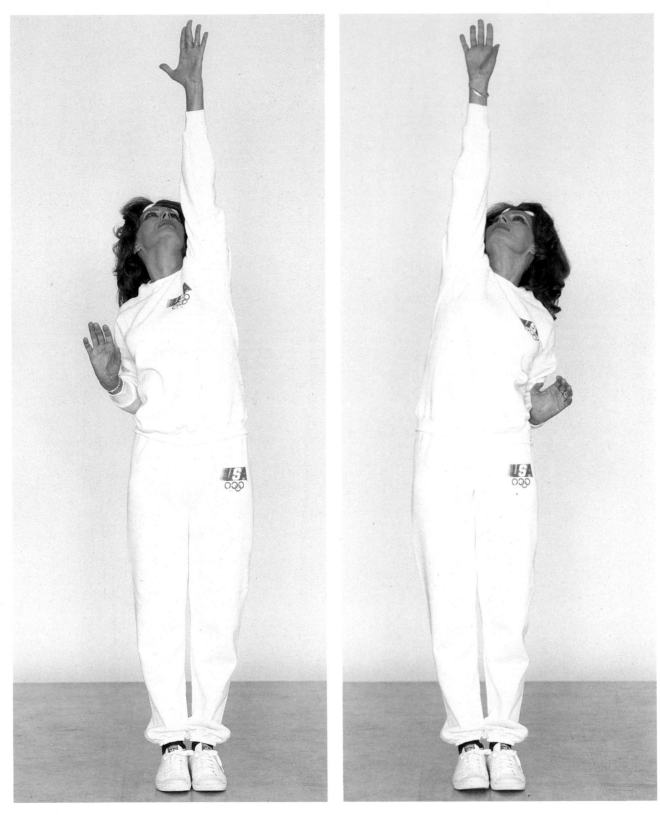

ARM REACH   Reach slowly upward with one hand until it is as high as you can get it. Hold the position for a few seconds. Repeat with the other hand. This stretches the waist and sides as well as the arms.

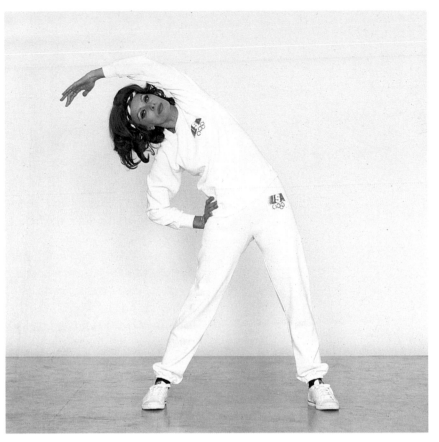

SIDE STRETCH   Stand with your feet apart. Put your right hand on your waist and your left arm over your head. Slowly reach to the right side until you feel the stretch on your left. Hold this position for a few seconds. Reverse the position of your hands and bend to the other side. I do this three or four times on each side.

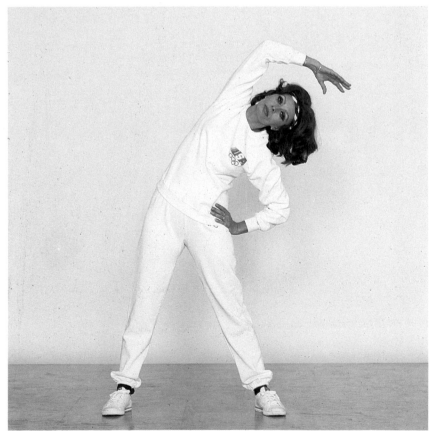

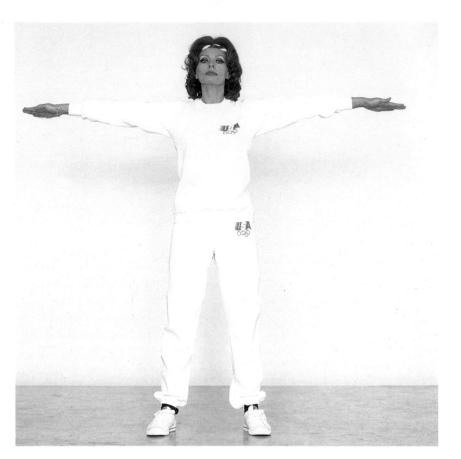

ARM CIRCLES   Extend your arms to your sides at shoulder height. Circle them slowly forward, beginning with small circles and gradually making them larger (I do about ten circles). Then circle your arms backward, starting with large circles and ending with small ones. Because I am especially concerned about having firm arms, I always do this exercise. It is also good for the chest.

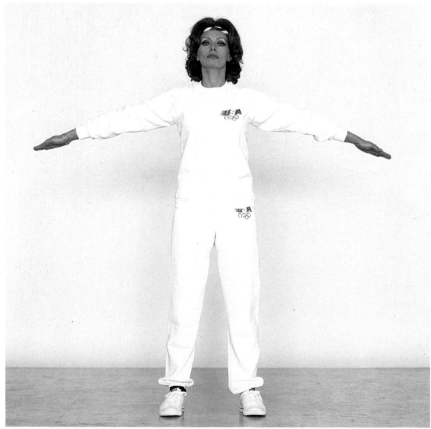

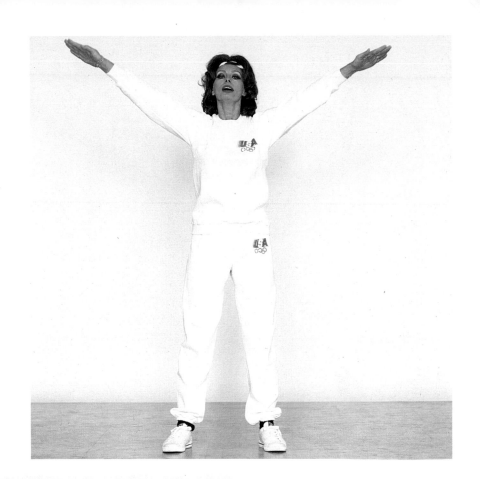

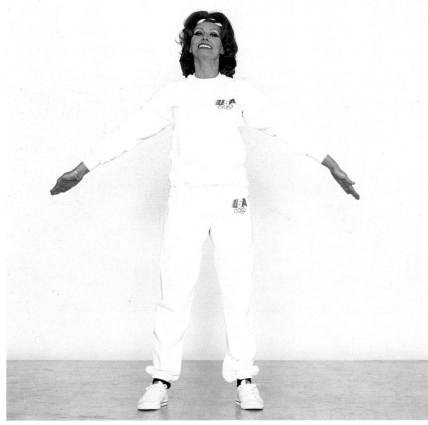

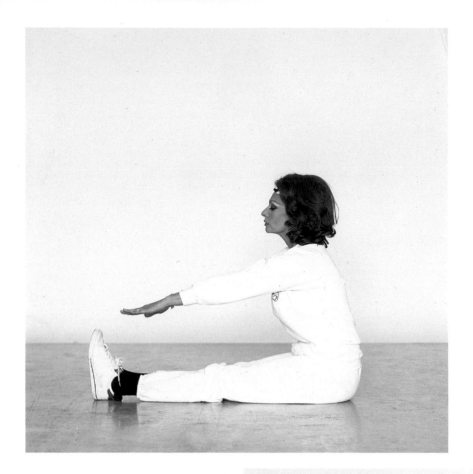

LEG STRETCH   Sit on the floor with your legs in front of you. Bend your left leg, bringing your left foot as close as you can to your body. Now, keeping your right leg straight, reach forward with both hands and hold your right ankle or foot. Go as far down as you can without straining – remember you are stretching. Eventually you will be able to rest your body along your leg, a feat I manage once or twice a week. Hold your lowered position for a few seconds, and then reverse legs and repeat. You will find that this exercise stretches your legs and your back.

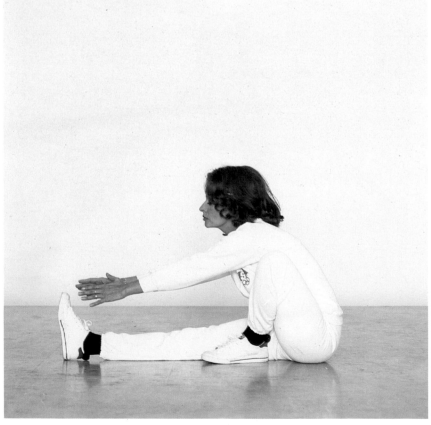

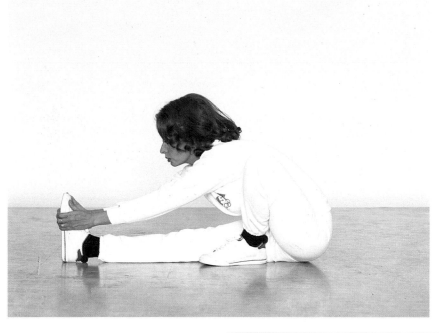

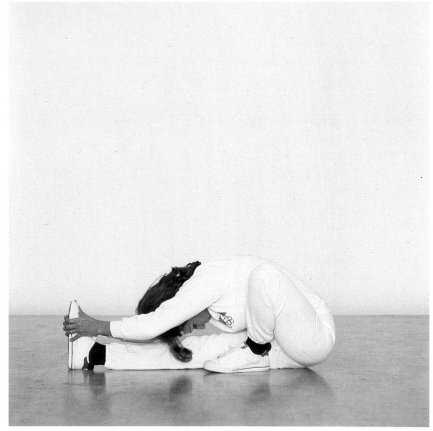

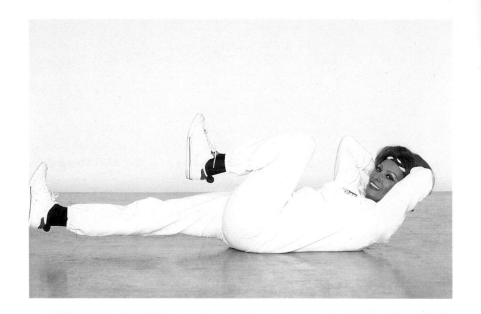

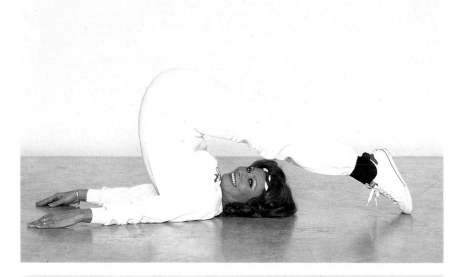

Some more advanced exercises for particular problem areas. Top: Pedaling with the feet flexed is great for the tummy muscles. Centre: This, a yoga relaxation position, demands suppleness but it opens up the shoulders and gives a good stretch to the thighs. (Note: You must not let your spine sag, and should never do this exercise when menstruating.) Below: This version of the splits is also very good for toning the thighs.

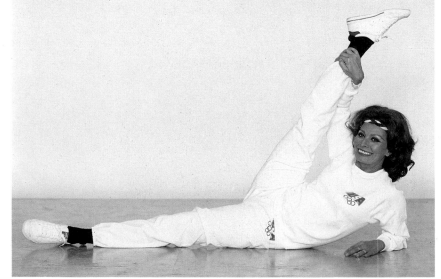

In the ten or fifteen minutes it takes me to do some of these stretches, I find that my mind has been set on a positive note because I have accomplished something even though I have only been up for a short while. Besides giving a feeling of accomplishment, these stretches also make me more aware of my body so that I believe they improve my posture throughout the day and help me to move more gracefully.

I should say that as well as doing these particular stretches every morning, I am also very conscious of stretching throughout the day. If I am reading, I take regular breaks and stretch to the ceiling. If I am working on a film, I always make a point of doing a few stretches between takes. Not only do they take the kinks out of my body, they also relieve tension to a remarkable degree.

Walking

As I mentioned before, aerobic exercise routines bore me and I have never been interested in sports, so years ago I adopted the simplest and best exercise in the world: walking. I know that it may not seem very fashionable these days when women lift weights and run marathons. Such activities are fine if they interest you, but not for someone like me. For one thing, because of my schedule, which changes constantly, I find it very difficult to block out time for a regular routine, and I know myself well enough to realize that if I started such a program I would just give it up eventually and feel defeated.

This brings me to one of the most wonderful things about walking: you can always do it, anywhere. You need no equipment except your feet and comfortable shoes, and you can fit it into any schedule. Walking gives you a chance to enjoy the weather, get to know your neighborhood or, if you are traveling, see a new place. I always find it exhilarating and enjoyable.

I was pleased to read recently of an experiment done in the United States involving various kinds of exercise. Groups of people were started on different exercise programs – some ran, some did calisthenics, some swam and some walked. At the end of the allotted time, they found that those people who walked had gained the most benefit. They lost the most weight and showed the most improvement in the condition of their hearts. The main reason seemed to be that none of them gave up. Some of the people doing the other exercises became discouraged, some were injured, some were just bored. But the people who were walking did it every day and even took pleasure in it. I think that, after all, results are what matter in an exercise program.

Did you know that you burn as many calories when you walk a mile as when you run it? Of course, it takes longer but it still works. Even before I knew that, I had decided walking would be my major aerobic activity.

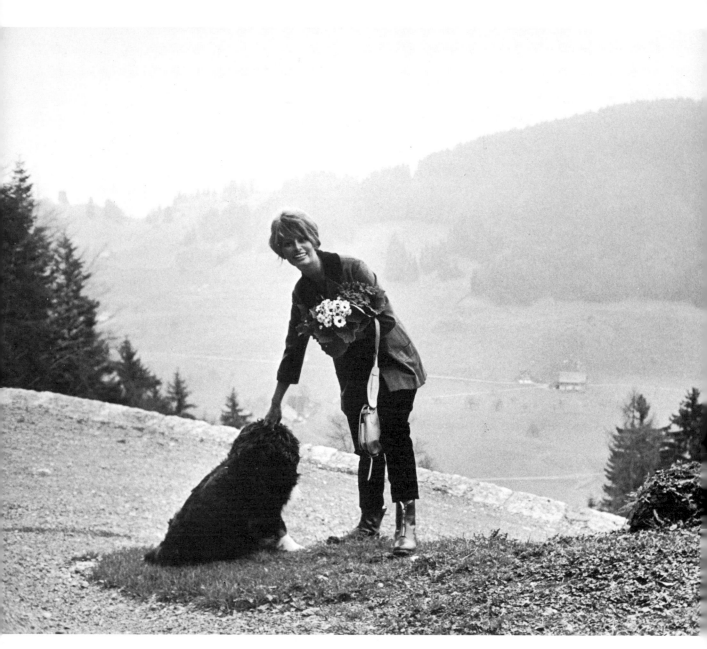

Enjoying the mountain air on one of my long walks near my home in Switzerland.

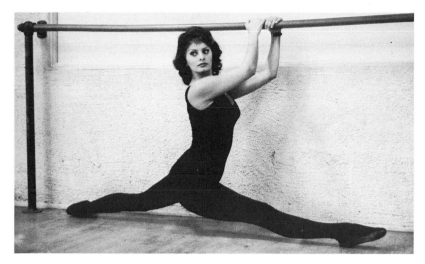

Practicing the splits for my role in Heller in Pink Tights.

"Aerobic" is the key word: it means exercise that raises the heartbeat enough to get more blood (and therefore more oxygen) pumped through the system. If you just stroll down the street, window shopping, it won't have this effect. You must walk fast enough and long enough to get your heart working – usually fifteen minutes is the minimum. I usually try to walk for about an hour every other day. I try not to carry too much because additional weight can throw your posture off balance. When I am staying at my house in Bürgenstock in Switzerland, I walk for hours at a time. I just take off on a trail in the snow or through the woods, and walk at a brisk pace until I realize that people at home will start to worry, and then I turn around. Now that the boys are bigger, they often come with me and we have great fun.

If you don't take any other exercise, why not try walking? It is so easy to do. If you take it seriously, you will find that there are many ways to work it into your day. Sometimes it is just a matter of getting off the bus sooner or parking your car a distance from your destination so you have to walk there. Maybe you should leave the car at home entirely. I am sure that if you think about it you will have good ideas of when and where to walk.

Trouble Spots

Every woman has certain parts of her body that need special attention either because of weakness or flabbiness. For that reason, walking alone isn't enough to keep you in good shape. I have a group of specific exercises that I do for these trouble spots, and I will share them with you. These exercises won't make you lose weight, but they will make your muscles stronger and firmer. I do them about three times a week, either in the morning after I do my stretching exercises, or later in the day before a bath or shower.

TUMMY The tummy is a big trouble area for women. If you don't exercise to keep your abdominal muscles firm, your stomach will stick out. Girdles make the problem worse because if you rely on them, you never use your muscles. Bad posture can make even a flat stomach protrude, so remember to stand with your stomach tucked in at all times. Just by doing that, you strengthen your muscles.

Here are my tummy exercises:

1. Lie on your back with your knees bent and your feet flat on the floor. Curling your back forward and using your stomach muscles, sit up as far as you can. Lower yourself to the floor. I do this about eight times.

2. Sit on the floor with your legs straight out in front of you and your hands resting on the floor behind your back. Lean back slightly, keeping your back rounded, and lift your legs about a foot above the floor. Pedal as if you were on a bicycle, being sure to extend your leg fully every time. I do this about ten times.

THIGHS Even if you walk regularly, it is hard to keep your thighs firm. These exercises will help.

1. Stand next to a table or chair and hold on to it with your left hand for support. Extend your right leg and bend your left knee as much as you can until you have lowered your body about a foot toward the floor. Hold this position for a count of five. Repeat with the left leg extended. Do this with each leg about three times.

2. Lie on your back with your arms extended at your sides at shoulder level. Bring your left knee up to your chest, then straighten your leg toward the ceiling, keeping your foot flexed. Slowly lower the left leg across your right leg until it touches the floor, keeping your shoulders on the floor. Lift your leg up again until it points to the ceiling, then, keeping it straight, lower it to the floor. Repeat with the other leg. I do this five times with each leg.

UPPER ARMS Most women find that their upper arms are among the first places to show lack of muscle tone.

1. Stand with your elbows bent and your palms resting on the middle of your upper back. Lift one arm and point it toward the ceiling. Bring that arm back to the starting position. Repeat with the other arm. I do this about fifteen times with each arm.

2. Stand with your feet together and bend forward at the waist, keeping your back straight. Bend your knees so that you are not putting too much strain on your back. Bring your elbows up, pressing them close to your sides and bending them so your forearms are perpendicular to the floor. Bring your arms up behind you and then slowly back to the bent position, pressing in hard all the time. Repeat this about six times.

BOTTOM   If you wear slacks as often as I do, you will want to have a trim bottom. Unfortunately, we don't seem to use the relevant muscles enough in the course of an average day, so here is what I recommend to strengthen and tone them.

1. Stand with your right hand holding the back of a chair or a table for support. Raise your left leg with the knee bent until your foot is about a foot from the floor. With your knee bent, push the thigh forward and hold in this position for a count of five. Then push your thigh back behind your body as far as you can and hold it, again for a count of five. Do this about eight times with each leg.

2. Stand with your right hand on the back of a chair. Bring your left leg out to the side, foot raised so only your toes touch the floor. Keeping your toes on the floor, move your foot until it is behind your right leg. Still keeping your toes on the floor, return the leg to its starting position. Do this about eight times with each leg.

LOWER BACK   Women often have problems with their backs; usually this is because their abdominal and hip muscles aren't strong enough. Here is an exercise I do to keep my back limber. Be sure to stop doing any exercise if you feel that it is straining your back, and if you have a history of back trouble I suggest you check with your doctor before you do any exercises for your back.

1. Lie on your back with your knees bent and your feet flat on the floor near your bottom. Bring your knees up and as close to your chest as possible. Use your hands to grab your knees and bring them close, then lift your head and try to touch your forehead to your knees. Lower your head and legs to the starting position. I do this, sometimes along with my morning stretches, about eight times.

The Mystery of Beauty

CHARM:
ITS MYSTERY AND TECHNIQUE

*T*he glint in Clark Gable's eyes. Marcello Mastroianni's engaging openness. Katharine Hepburn's courage. Marilyn Monroe's vulnerability. These qualities attract and delight us. We notice them and want to be with the person who has them. We react to them as if to a magic spell; we are mesmerized. This is charm.

Charm is the "invisible" part of beauty. No one who is totally lacking in it can be beautiful. At the same time, no woman, no matter how beautiful, will draw people to her and enjoy the benefits of beauty if she is completely devoid of charm. The magic of this quality is that it can make a plain woman uniquely appealing. Charm dissolves a multitude of physical imperfections. Beauty gets you noticed, intelligence and wit demand recognition, but charm will make you memorable.

Why even discuss charm? Well, if you go to some trouble to be beautiful, as I think you should, it is a good idea to keep in mind why you do it. You want to be beautiful for your own satisfaction, yes, but you also want to find love and friendship, perhaps to achieve success, and certainly to please the people around you. Just being pretty won't accomplish much, but when you add the power of charm, you will be hard to resist.

I am devoting this attention to charm because I think it is too often neglected as an element of beauty. You can buy the very best clothes, have your hair done in the perfect style, apply your makeup with a sure hand, but still, without charm, you are like a mannequin. I am not saying that charm is a device you can arbitrarily add to your life in order to attain a certain goal: you can't just put it on for dinner parties or for a night out on the town. Charm is like good weather – it affects every minute of every day we spend with others. A captivating woman is a delight to have around because she makes everything more fun. She adds sparkle to any occasion, whether it's a walk in the woods, a phone conversation or a formal gathering. A charming woman is one who remembers birthdays or writes wonderful thank-you notes or is thoughtful in her own special way. Charm can be as straightforward as sending a gift to a friend who is sick. It can be as whimsical as a spontaneous invitation to a bike ride. It can be as subtle as a smile of

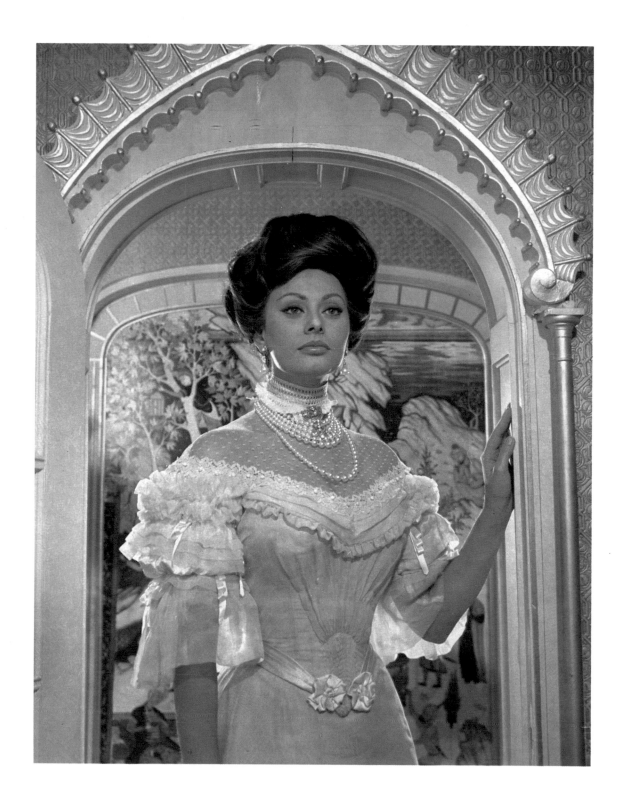

recognition. Charm has many guises and is not limited to any one quality.

When I remember John Wayne, I don't think of the big macho cowboy of legend, although that is what I expected before I met him. We starred together in a film called *Legend of the Lost,* much of which was shot on location in the Sahara Desert. It was broiling hot by day and cold at night, and one night the gas heater in my room tipped over and I almost died from carbon monoxide poisoning. Through all this, John Wayne was polite but distant. Then one day when we were walking through the sand (it seems as if we were always walking through the sand!), John gave me something. It felt cold and heavy in my hand, but when I held it up I realized that it was a desert rose – a rock formation that occurs in the desert and looks very much like a full-blown rose. It was a soft pink color, and very beautiful. I don't know if he had just found it – they weren't particularly common in that area – or if he had saved it from another outing. I was so touched by this gesture that I could never again take seriously the image of the rough, tough John Wayne. For me he became a man of charm and sensitivity.

I used to think that charm was something you were born with or did without. Some people seemed to be charming without effort; others seemed to have no special power to attract at all. The charming ones, I thought, were just lucky. The others would have to work much harder for what they wanted. It wasn't until I began my acting career that my eyes were opened on this subject.

All the characters I have played in films have been charming. To be honest, this isn't because I am so bewitching, but simply because filmmakers know that audiences will be more interested in watching beguiling people on the screen than dull ones. But don't think for a minute that charm automatically goes with fancy clothes and money. Yes, in the movie *Arabesque,* for example, I play a woman who is rich and elegant and has a very polished, sophisticated quality. But in *A Special Day* my appeal is of a totally different nature. I play a woman lost in the drudgery of her days, without money or time, but who still has her own natural charm.

So where does this elusive quality come from? When working in films, one learns that there are certain elements – gestures, looks, movements – that help create a character on the screen. There is a technique and an art to charm. At the same time, we have all seen films in which an actor or actress fails to create the illusion of charm. So it is not all in the technique. There is something else.

I believe that in addition to technique, charm demands honesty. True charm is an honest expression of self. Marcello Mastroianni's honesty, which is often disarming, is not technique. It is a part of his personality and character, and it enchants everyone. Sometimes a certain boldness or shyness or even a faux pas can be charming because they seem to come

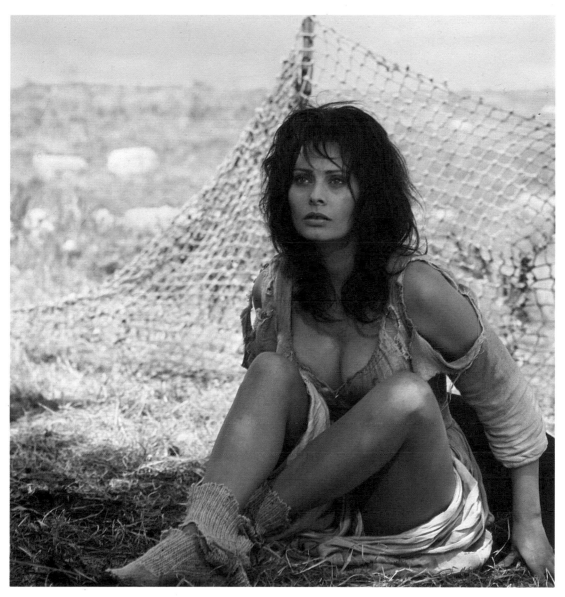

I try to discover the particular charm of each character I play. Here I am as Aldonza, the serving maid in Man of La Mancha.

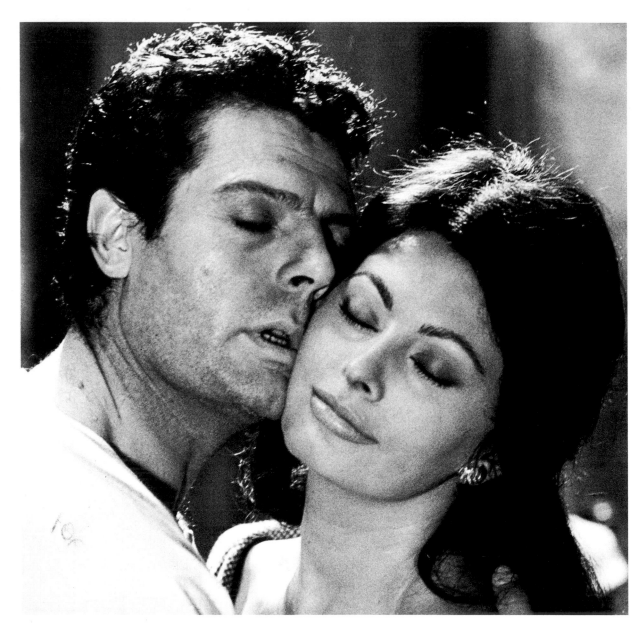

A romantic pose with Marcello Mastroianni in Yesterday, Today and Tomorrow, *1963.*

from the soul, they are completely honest, and they allow us to see a special side of someone.

It is not always easy to be oneself. It can demand a certain kind of courage. If, for example, you are with people who are music experts but you know nothing about music, it is very tempting simply to nod along, pretending to knowledge that you don't have. Much better to admit that you are ignorant of the subject, and that you are delighted to have the opportunity to learn more. This seems simple but it is not so easy to do, for we always have such a desire to impress others and to protect ourselves.

When I speak of charm as growing from honesty, I recommend that you not be too literal about it. Chattering about your defects and proclaiming all those things you know nothing about can be numbingly boring. The point is to recognize what is true about yourself and express it freely. If you are shy, don't pretend to be the life of the party. If you are a bad dancer, don't spend the night stepping on people's toes. But if you are proud of your ability to sing, don't pretend otherwise. Charm comes when you reveal a unique side of yourself to others.

There is one final element: in addition to honesty and technique, there is no charm without mystery. Now, I can't tell you how to be mysterious. But when you think about charm, you will realize that there is something about it that cannot be defined. Its mystery comes often in what is not said. It may be a certain look, a touch of the hand, an implication that there is something more than what appears to the eye. As I have said, there is no point in consciously trying to become "mysterious." But I do think that it is helpful to remember that when we try to be charming, there is great power in what we imply as well as in what we do.

When I first met the man who had written the screenplay of *Woman of the River,* I knew that he had already been involved in the production of two other films for which I had been passed over, and I thought he was hostile to me. He was waiting in a deserted room, listening to a mambo on the radio. I wanted to do something that expressed a part of myself that I couldn't put into words; so impulsively, I leaped into the room and, dancing the mambo, approached him. I learned later that this man wasn't hostile to me at all. When we became close friends, he told me that that strange dance was one of the most charming things he had ever seen.

Charm is an individual quality. To be charming you need only concentrate on your special assets and how you can present them to others. You have to be honest in expressing yourself. When others sense that they are seeing a true expression of your personality, they will be charmed.

Only you can tell what is unique and charming about yourself. Perhaps it is your smile, your laugh, your kindness. Perhaps it is the way you see the funny side of life. Perhaps it is your serenity. Whatever your particular appeal, it cannot help but be enhanced by the techniques of charm.

The effects of charm are felt only in our relations with other people. And it is often the small things that we do for others that make the difference.

I remember the first time I met Charlie Chaplin. I was in England, staying in a rented cottage in Ascot, and he was to come and show me the script for *A Countess from Hong Kong.* The meeting had been arranged in advance and I was terribly nervous. Charlie Chaplin had been a hero of my childhood. Watching his antics on the screeen I could forget the war and the poverty that was all around me in Pozzuoli. I felt a great gratitude toward him and was very much in awe of his talent.

When I heard the doorbell ring I smoothed my dress and took a deep breath. And there before me was the small giant with a bouquet of flowers in his hand. I was charmed. That small gesture, the spring flowers, broke the ice and made us both feel at ease. It was such a simple gesture and, after all, not exactly unique, but it set things on the right path. Ultimately we became good friends and knowing him was an experience I will always treasure.

The point of my story is the bouquet: it worked the magic of charm. And it shows how little things can smooth the way between people. I think we would all do well to remember these little tthings – manners, warmth, sympathy – in our encounters with others. What may begin as a technique becomes a habit and, eventually, charm.

Manners

Social occasions are opportunities for pleasure and stimulation. Charm can ease the way, but it is important to pay some attention to manners because they are the framework upon which charm is built. I know people without manners, and although I might come to think of them as interesting, I will never find them charming.

Sometimes manners, like horseless carriages, seem to be an idea whose time has come and gone. Today's culture is so informal and so flexible that we tend to think manners are outmoded and that common sense will serve us better. I think this is a big mistake. There are many structured situations in which an accepted form of behavior will ease the way. Indeed, manners can and should affect every transaction we make throughout every day of our lives. They can make the difference between a cheerful existence and a miserable one. Every exchange you have with another person is touched by manners, good or bad. Whether you are dealing with your mother or a cabdriver, your manners will affect the tone of the exchange.

Manners are really about graciousness, the quality that makes others feel at ease. If you keep that in mind, you will understand why they are important. Once you know the structure of manners, you will feel at home

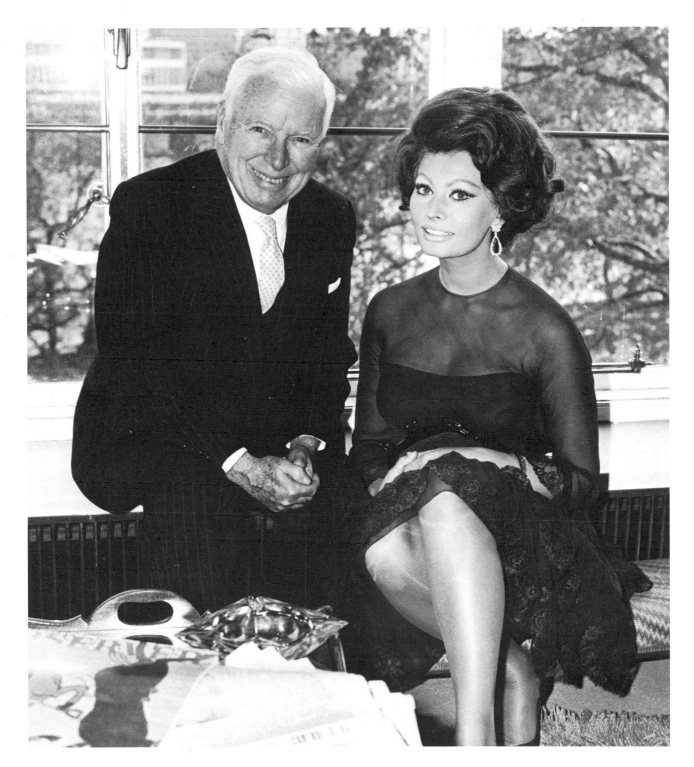

Preparing for A Countess from Hong Kong *with my dear friend Charlie Chaplin, master of charm.*

anywhere in the world and you will be able to make others feel that way too.

I have had many varied experiences in many different social situations, and I have noticed what a big difference good manners can make. Sometimes I get an instant bad impression of someone because of their manners. Usually people are gracious to me because of who I am, but I notice when they are rude or unkind to others whom they think are unimportant. When I see this, I take an instant dislike to those people. I never show it or say anything, but from that moment on, I think differently of them.

Study correct manners if you don't feel comfortable with what you already know. Read a book on etiquette and observe the behavior of those who seem able to make you and everyone else comfortable on social occasions. I do not suggest that you make a career of learning manners, but everyone can use a refresher course now and again. And if you are a mother, you have a big responsibility to teach your children manners. The home is the place to learn them. If your children grow up with good manners, their lives will be much easier.

There are certain everyday occasions that give you an opportunity to display good manners. An important one is when you are introducing strangers. So often people in the street or at parties simply announce the names of those introduced, which gives no opportunity for them to sail into conversation. They end up staring at each other and feeling uncomfortable. I am especially aware of this when I am introduced to people who may know who I am but I don't know anything about them. I would like to have a conversational opening so that I could learn something about them. It makes such a difference to say, "This is Maria, who has just returned from her first trip to Hong Kong," or "This is John, who has just become a father." Suddenly the opportunities are limitless. Making that kind of introduction at a party, and being certain to introduce every person to someone the moment he or she arrives, will ensure that everyone feels at home from the start. Of course, it takes more trouble on your part to do this, and you have to know something to say about each guest, but that is one of the most important duties of a hostess. Good food and wine mean nothing if your guests do not feel at home.

Conversation

Conversation is the soul of a party or any kind of social get-together. Good conversation grows from an interest in learning about others. Many people think that being a good conversationalist means telling lots of witty stories and being the center of attention. This isn't true at all. Clever anecdotes add spice but they are not the real meat of conversation. It is just as important to

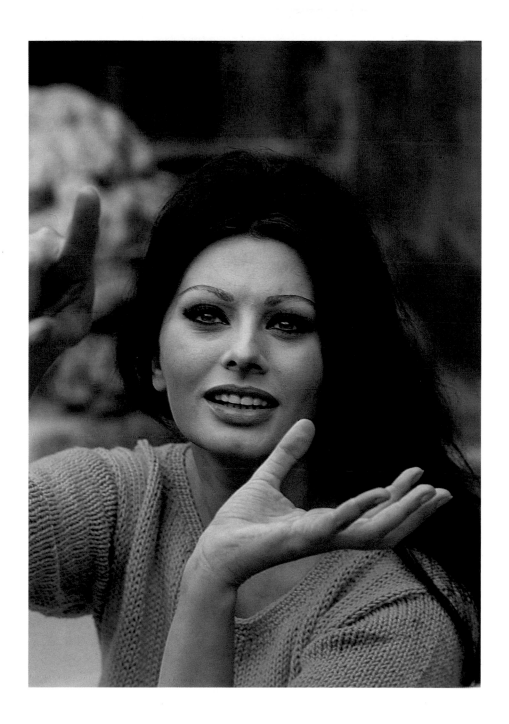

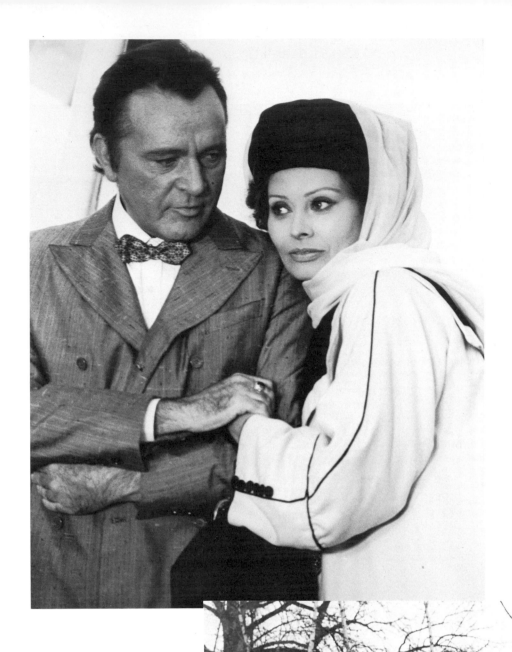

On the set of The Voyage *with Richard Burton (above), and talking with Noël Coward during the shooting of* Lady L.

listen as to talk. Conversation is an exchange, and there can be no exchange if one person is doing all the talking.

Richard Burton is an excellent conversationalist. I met him in the summer of 1973 when he stayed at my house in Marino. We were scheduled to star together in Vittorio de Sica's *The Voyage,* and Richard wanted to get away from the photographers and the press and relax before the filming began. We had wonderful long conversations about everything you can think of. Richard is a fiercely intelligent man. He quotes literature, uses ancient history to bolster his points and has such a broad frame of reference that I envy him. He never resorts to gossip and is really more interested in talking about ideas than people, which is another quality I admire. (Of course, he isn't perfect. After countless games, he has never beaten me at Scrabble. Like Peter O'Toole, who has also gone down to bitter defeat at my hands.)

Do you ever worry that once you are among other people you will have nothing to say? Some people are so glib and extroverted that they can't imagine this ever happening to them. For the rest of us, including me, some preparation can ease the way. As you shower or put on makeup, give a bit of thought to what subjects you might introduce. This may sound contrived, but I think it is only common sense. In fact, even though I have never heard anyone recommend this preparation, I suspect that lots of people do it all the time. A newspaper article that you have just read, a book you disliked, the role of animals in one's life – any subject can get things rolling and rescue a conversational lull.

On occasion, you may meet famous or accomplished people. If you are so fortunate, you should first make an effort to learn something about them and what they have achieved. Don't do this in order to flatter or impress that person because this attitude will simply make you both uncomfortable. But by knowing something about them and their work, you will be able to open a conversation, make them feel at ease, and, at the same time, perhaps learn something else valuable.

When I was filming *Lady L,* I heard that Noël Coward was coming to visit the set, which was at a famous castle in Yorkshire. The truth is, I didn't know much about him. But I learned all I could in the time available, and when he arrived I was able to talk to him about his life and experiences. Afterward I read two of his plays and I liked them so much that I was really sorry I hadn't had a chance to read them in advance so we could have discussed them too.

In Defense of Shyness

Before we leave the party, I must say something in defense of shyness. I myself am shy and I know what it is like to enter a room full of strangers and

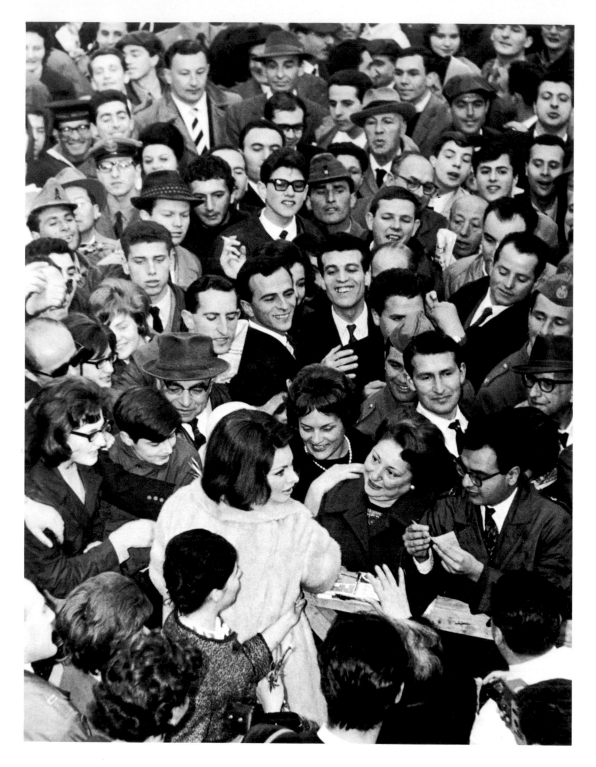

I am always grateful to my fans, but it takes a lot of self-control and training to keep your composure in a situation like this.

feel an attack of nerves as all eyes turn to look. You might not believe this, given my career and my work, but it is true. I don't like going to fancy parties, but I do so because I understand the obligation I have to the public that made me famous. I think it is foolish for actors to disdain their public. In any case, when I go to such events I am usually prepared. But one night, when I was in London filming *The Millionairess,* I went to the Savoy Hotel with Peter Sellers for dinner. As we entered the dining room, I realized suddenly that every eye was upon us. My knees got so weak that I began to sink to the floor and only Peter's support – he saw me blanch – kept me from falling down. I can handle the spotlight when I am expecting it because I feel the right kind of tension that gives me strength, but when it hits me without warning I turn into a jellyfish.

There is nothing wrong with being shy and it is nothing to be ashamed of. The trick is to conquer your shyness in a graceful way. Some people cope with it by retreating entirely and isolating themselves. Others become clowns or bores in a misguided attempt to distract people from their shyness. Neither of these approaches works. I remember when I was filming *The Fall of the Roman Empire,* one of my costars had a kind of aggressiveness that was turning the cast and crew against him. I recognized that underneath his obnoxious pose, he was really shy and I believed that he was a good person. I took him aside and said, "I don't think you are really a rude person, so don't confuse people with that kind of behavior." This remark may just have made him think again about his approach, for he gradually relaxed and won the support of the rest of the cast.

I never try to be aggressively sociable because it is not my nature and I wouldn't be effective. I make a point of selecting someone I can talk with who makes me feel comfortable, and then I focus my attention on that person. In this way I do not have to cope with a large group of people but I am still involved in the party. This is much easier and, for me at least, it is more rewarding.

It is important if you are shy to train yourself to be able to enjoy a party even if, given the choice, you would rather be at home alone with a book. There are times when you need the company of others, and you should savor the opportunities to meet new people and expand your horizons. You must approach a party with a positive attitude. Convince yourself that you are going to have a good time and you will. Don't isolate yourself in a corner where no one will feel any inclination to talk to you. Don't enter a room as if you wished to be anywhere else but there. On the other hand, don't think that it is sophisticated to act bored and superior. Be confident that you have something to offer another person, and your confidence will create an aura that will draw others to you.

Voice and Gestures

I once heard that Charlie Chaplin had said of me, "What can you expect of a girl raised halfway between a gun factory and an erupting volcano?" When I first started in films, I was self-conscious about my voice so I assumed he was referring to that. I was mortified. What a relief to learn that he was describing my temperament!

As an actress, I am very conscious of the sound and inflection of voices because the voice is an instrument of the craft of acting. Have you ever sat in a restaurant or on a bus and suddenly heard one voice above all the rest? It was probably especially loud or strident. This teaches you almost all you need to know about voices, for it seems we notice them only when they are unattractive. If the voice is pleasing, you are not aware of it: only the words impress you.

A simple way to listen to your own voice is to open a magazine, put your nose right into the center and say a few words. Your voice will echo back, and you will get a good idea of what you sound like to others. (I suggest that you try this when you are alone!) You can also use a tape recorder to get some sense of how you sound to others. You will probably be surprised to find that you can hardly recognize your own voice. It is a good idea to tape yourself when you are having a casual conversation with a friend. When you play it back you will notice inflections and speech rhythms that you were never aware of. You may find that you have some bad speech habits – perhaps you repeat certain words, maybe you speak too fast. You can learn a lot from a ten-minute tape.

When I began my career, I needed to learn to lower my voice. It was very high-pitched and, in fact, it was even irritating to my own ears. I grew to hate the sound of it, so I decided that something must be done. I set about lowering my voice. With lots of discipline my natural speaking tone became lower than it used to be, and when I act in a film, it is lower still.

There is something about a voice in a low register that is far more pleasing to the ear than a high-pitched one. A low voice also has more authority. I am sure you have noticed this on television: when two people are arguing a point, the one whose voice becomes high and excited loses the sympathy of listeners even if they in fact agree with the point he or she is making. The one who remains calm, with a low, deliberate voice – that is the person who wins our confidence. This is something worth remembering when you feel the impulse to argue with someone. If you must have an argument, you might as well win your point, and a low, calm voice will be a strong ally.

Perhaps I am particularly aware of this problem of voice control because as a Neapolitan I have a fiery temper. When I lose it, my voice becomes

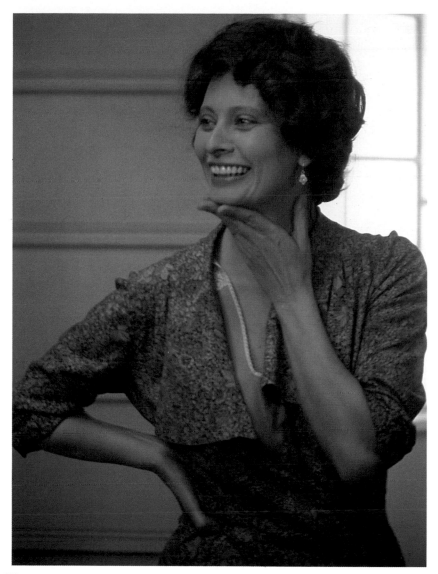

When I played the role of an aging housewife in A Special Day, *I adopted the gestures which I thought brought out her particular appeal.*

something that no one would want to hear for long. One of these days I hope I will learn completely to control my temper, but until I succeed I will at least try to keep my voice as calm and low as possible.

When considering self-expression, especially in connection with charm, we must not neglect gestures and movements. These are as personal as a signature, and they can be very charming when they are graceful and appropriate. They can amplify what we are saying and help us to be calm when we are nervous.

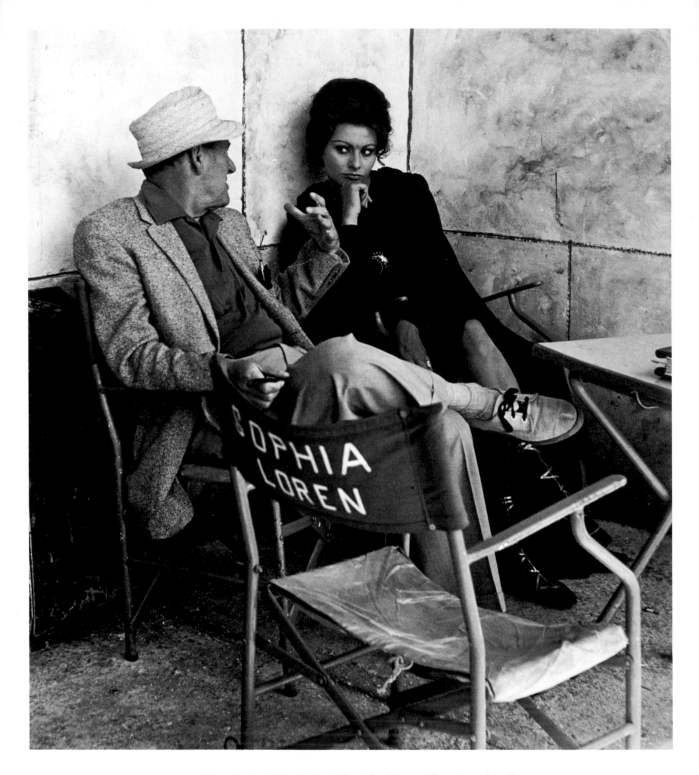

A break in filming The Fall of the Roman Empire *with director Anthony Mann in Madrid, 1964.*

While I wouldn't suggest that you put great effort into changing your natural gestures, you should be aware of them in case there are occasions when you would like to alter the impression you give. Controlled gestures create an aura of authority and calm. This can be very useful, especially when you are in a situation which you find difficult. You will also discover that by disciplining your body to remain in repose you will actually feel more calm and more in control. I have found this useful to remember in television appearances when I want both to conquer my nerves and also to avoid distracting my listeners with lots of hand movements.

Warmth and Humor

Perhaps the real soul of charm is personal warmth. We all know certain people who seem sympathetic and caring, and how pleasurable it is to be with them. Others are afraid to show affection or be warm, and this, in my opinion, is a great tragedy. For men in particular, this can be a problem, and they should work very hard to overcome it.

Of course, there are ways of showing warmth other than by a physical touch or embrace. Appreciation that is shown with a note or a small remembrance can be very touching. If you are grateful for something that someone has done for you, don't simply think about it – let that person know. And do it quickly. A brief note sent promptly is often far more appreciated than a lavish gift that is late in coming.

I believe humor is certainly a great part of charm. I suppose a sense of humor is the one thing that my friends have in common. The sound of laughter is so beautiful and refreshing. Hearing children laugh is like listening in on heaven.

Humor also allows people to share thoughts and ideas in a very happy way. Like music, it is a common ground where strangers can meet and become friends. You may think that you have nothing in common with someone until you find that you can share a joke. Some of the most wonderful friendships are built on nothing more or less than a shared sense of humor. When I was working on *The Pride and the Passion* with Cary Grant and Frank Sinatra, there was much joking on the set. My English was so primitive that I didn't catch many of the jokes, but because I wanted to join in I would try to laugh at the right times. I had an Italian friend there who understood my predicament, and once he caught my eye while I was laughing with the others. In that moment we realized that we were both laughing at nothing, and that made us only laugh harder. From then on, each time the others shared a joke, we would laugh the hardest because we were laughing at ourselves. Certainly without humor life would be terribly dull.

MEN AND LOVE

*P*eople are always asking me about the men in my past. What was it like to work with Gregory Peck? Is Paul Newman really so handsome? What about Frank Sinatra and Marlon Brando? Did you find them attractive? Many people, especially women, consider me lucky because in my work I have met and continue to meet the most fascinating and handsome screen actors in the world. Men who represent the dreams of so many women and the ambitions of so many boys are my colleagues and sometimes my friends.

Well, here is the real truth about what it is like to work with such stars. Think for a minute of your husband, your boyfriend or your father. Working with the giants of the screen world is very much like working with the men you know so well in your life. When you are with these actors day in and day out, sometimes feeling tired, sometimes irritable, the enchantment, the thrill, the powerful allure dissolve. Some days are great fun, others are sheer misery. With some of your co-workers you develop lasting friendships; with some you keep hoping that fate will never again require you to meet. I have talked about discipline. Well, it takes the strongest discipline to passionately kiss and caress a man you don't really like, making it seem as real as you can for an audience. Fortunately, that has only happened to me a few times.

To say these men have ordinary qualities is not intended to diminish their greatness. When I am questioned about the actors with whom I have worked, I can't deny a pleasant feeling of pride and accomplishment. Just think! My leading men have included Cary Grant, Frank Sinatra, Marlon Brando, Marcello Mastroianni, Gregory Peck and Richard Burton. I could add Paul Newman, William Holden, Trevor Howard, Jean Gabin, Omar Sharif – but I do not want to slight so many others, so I will stop here. If I were asked to create the ideal man, it certainly would suffice to take a feature or a quality from each of these fabulous partners of mine. Here is how this composite creature would begin to shape up: he would have Paul's blue eyes, Marlon's sensual mouth, Gregory's finely shaped nose, Richard's vibrant voice, Cary's smart slenderness, Jean's magnetism, Marcello's charming and honest nature.

Now, before we lose ourselves to a creature of the imagination, I should tell you that I have often thought of such an ideal man, created him in my

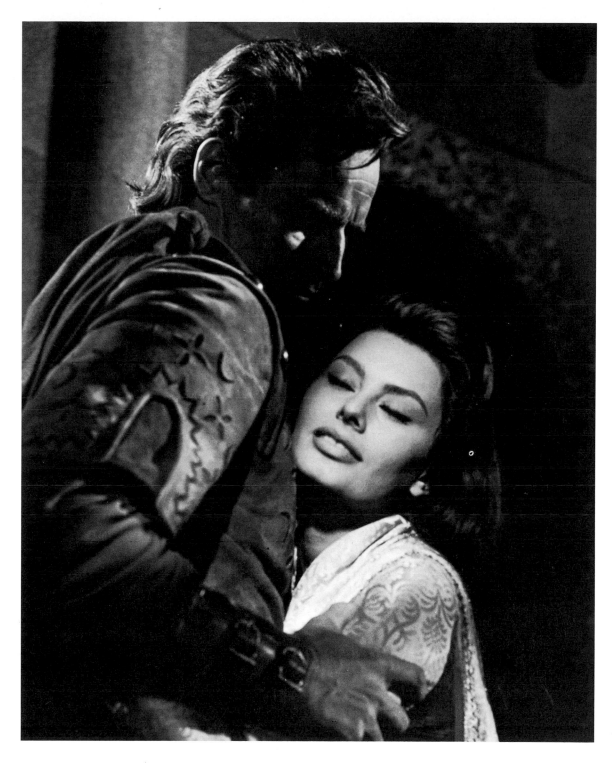

With Charlton Heston in El Cid.

mind's eye, and, in my opinion, he is a failure. A man who embodied all these qualities would be a disaster. In the first place he would be faultless, and what could be more monotonous than a man who does not provoke some healthy negative reaction? Who could live with a man who is so perfectly handsome, charming and imbued with the character of a saint?

Secondly, the ideal man is not an abstract phenomenon, independent from us. We women contribute to create a major portion of this ideal and we adapt it, as a coat made to measure, to the man we have chosen. That is why a woman will sometimes choose a man who seems, to all her friends at least, quite unsuitable. She sees something special in this man, something that perhaps really is there or perhaps is just in her eyes. Love may indeed be blind, as the saying goes, but even so it is important to have some measure of reality when you choose a man to love. If your eyes are completely clouded with a vision that you have made up from movie stars and other famous men, a vision that bears little resemblance to the real man, you are bound to be disappointed.

If we try to be realistic about the kind of man to love, we have to abandon the ideal composite that I built out of Paul and Cary and Marlon and others. Once we are past the dreamy stage of adolescence, we have no need for such a man. For a handsome face and a graceful figure will not satisfy a mature woman. She is ready for the real challenge of love that admits imperfection and ambiguity. So what I have to say to you about love is not about movie stars, it is about the man or men in your life – the one across the breakfast table or the one you are waiting to meet. That man, because he is right for you in some strange and unpredictable way, is not less than ideal, he is *your* ideal.

Love Under the Microscope

In sharing with you my thoughts about love, I can, of course, speak only from my own experience. But I think today we have become preoccupied with the idea of romantic love and its place in our lives. Perhaps it would do us all good to forget for a week, a month, a year about the health and vigor of our "relationships."

In the past, when people were engrossed in the urgent demands of daily life – finding food, building shelter, tending children and so on – they had less time to worry about the meaning of love in their lives. Love probably had more to do with survival than with self-realization. A good husband was one who provided well for his family. A wife didn't think about "quality time" with her husband. They were two people joined in a common pursuit, sometimes happy, sometimes straining at their yoke.

Today all that has changed. You are encouraged to expect that love will be the central adventure of your life. Love, when at last it happens, will change everything. You will have found that one person who will be your perfect partner, your better half. But isn't it curious that for people who have such esteem for love, such dependence upon love as an essential for happiness, such unbounded faith in the powers of love, we cannot stay in love for very long? It almost seems as if we are infatuated with love. Or indeed, that we like the idea of love better than its reality.

We probably all know an example of the young couple beginning a life together against adversity and deprivation. With little or no money, their life is simple and sometimes quite hard. But they share a goal. Whether they are working to become doctors, lawyers, artists, actors or good parents, they have a dream of what their future will be like. Then one or both of them achieves success and the dream unravels. Suddenly, everything seems different and they find they are no longer in love.

It is a familiar scenario and all too common in real life. The popular explanations are that one of them couldn't "handle" success, or wasn't "equal" to it, or hadn't "grown" quickly enough. I have my own explanation. When two people climb a hill together they do so hand in hand. But once they reach the top, they no longer quite know in which direction they want to go. Instead of standing side by side looking to the future, they tend to turn to each other and try to analyze the bond that joins them – a new bond because the old bond of the common goal is gone.

It is my opinion that love cannot bear relentless scrutiny. If we are constantly testing, examining, comparing, holding it up to the light, our love will weaken and eventually disappear. And yet today we are encouraged continually to weigh and study our love. Does he love me enough? In the right way – truly, exclusively, without reservation? Does he satisfy me sexually? Does he support my career? Does he admire my taste? Does he respect my friends? Does he truly share with me? Women's magazines are filled with such questions about love and marriage, and even include tests that we can take to see how our love compares with the accepted norm. It is as if we are all in competition to win an Oscar for the "Best and Most Perfect Relationship by This Year's Standards."

Love is private, solitary and unique. I know what I am talking about because constant scrutiny, not by myself but by the press, is a part of my life. I cherish my privacy and am dismayed by how eager journalists are to try to find something to report about me. I know I have chosen a life that puts me in the spotlight, and I am grateful to a public that is interested in me. But that doesn't alter my determination to keep my family life to myself as much as I can. I know that you, as a woman, can understand this, and if you are a mother, you will understand it even better.

Let us never forget that in order to dissect something, we must kill it first.

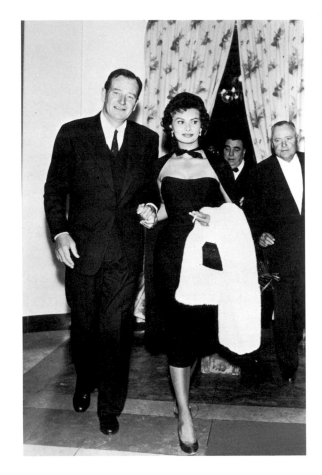

Some of my famous costars and
directors: John Wayne (right),
Marcello Mastroianni (far right),
Clark Gable (below), Charlie
Chaplin (centre) and Vittorio de
Sica (below, right).

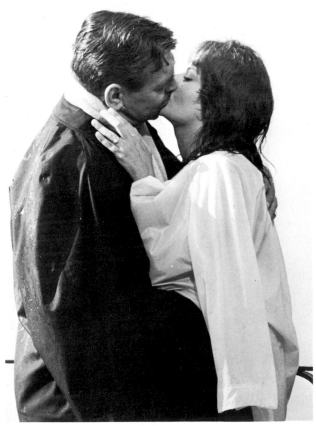

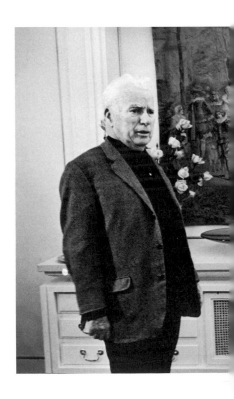

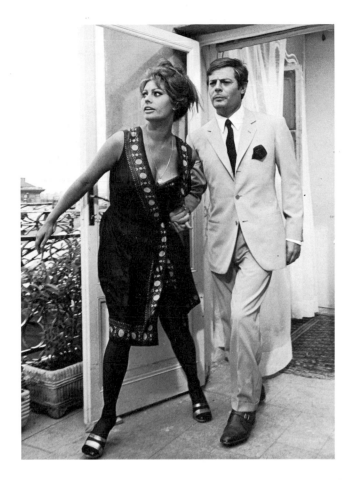

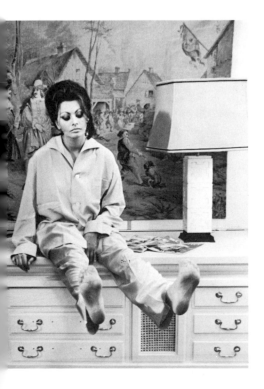

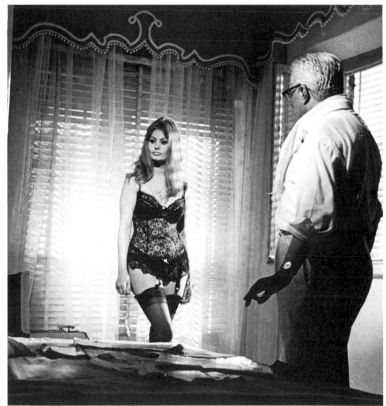

Love doesn't belong in a laboratory. It is haphazard by nature. It is more like a wildflower than a long-stemmed rose. It is shy, homely. Love should inspire and delight, but not really awe. If we transplant it, fertilize it, disturb it, it will probably die. With benign neglect and a warm atmosphere it will flourish and surprise us at every turn.

Love's Paradoxes

In order to find love, you must be disposed to love. You can't be like a princess in a castle waiting for someone to risk his life crossing the moat and scaling the wall. You must create a bridge and a ladder.

Pride is the greatest enemy of love because it closes your heart. It encourages you to compete. Once you think about love – real love and not a passing amusement – as a game, you have lost. There are always those moments when your pride makes you want to snap back, to have the last word. Let me tell you, although I know how hard it can be, that silence is better. You will ruin many wonderful moments in order to prove yourself.

And that's not all: when you make those comments or criticisms – ones you might regret later – you are often excited and your tone of voice is powerful. Your words will be convincing, perhaps more convincing than you know. As time goes by, these words will echo in your lover's mind and, like drops hitting a stone, eventually they will do their damage and there will be no repair. Those little bursts of pride which seem so justified at the moment will eventually destroy even the strongest love.

You must also recognize, as a mature adult, that trouble is a part of love. I think this takes time to learn. A young couple swings wildly from passion to revulsion. But as you grow wiser you come to realize that every cloud doesn't signal a hurricane. Some differences are worth a discussion, and sometimes an argument.

You certainly can have an argument or even a fight without destroying love. You must want to look beyond the fight, and if you both want this, you will achieve it. Perhaps this is one of the greatest values of marriage: it is a formal agreement that, if you value your promise, will carry you through the times when it may seem hopeless. And the more troubles you overcome, the more seasoned and understanding will your love become.

As a loving partner, you must not neglect the small things. The little matters of charm and kindness are the core of love. Too often you may forget them once you have won someone's heart. When you take love for granted and lose the desire to look and act your best for that person, the relationship will become strained and the joy will soon disappear.

When I was telling you about scent I mentioned the saying, "Love and perfume, you must not hoard." I will repeat it here. Love is not something to save, like an evening dress, for a special occasion. Love should be savored every day.

There is another virtue in cherishing the loving details of daily life: the more you do to express your love, the more love you will feel. If you spend the morning wondering why your lover didn't put his breakfast dish in the sink or why he never remembers your anniversary, I guarantee that you will be accumulating a reservoir of resentment. At the end of the day, you will be poised for new hurts and failings. Primed for disappointment, it is very likely that you will get what you are prepared for. If, on the other hand, you spend your time thinking about your lover's good points and doing things for your mutual pleasure, your good feelings will grow.

You come to love those you help. When you do something for someone, you feel a commitment to him and an investment in his well-being – you feel love. So it is a mistake to wait for love to grow without attention as if it were some magical force outside your control. It is no good waiting for that one special night, the night you put on your evening gown and feel love. You want to feel it all the time, and the way to achieve it is to do all the little things that nourish love and make it grow inside you.

Kindness Is the Soul of Love

You have probably heard Tolstoy's line "Happy families are all alike; every unhappy family is unhappy in its own way." I believe the common quality that happy families – and happy couples – share is kindness. Perhaps kindness sounds to you like a virtue for children – certainly it is not nearly as romantic as courage or honesty. But it is kindness that smooths the rough spots in a person's spirit.

Kindness can be expressed in so many ways. Sometimes it translates into silence. When your lover loses his keys for the fifth time that day, you have a right to be annoyed. Perhaps his mind is on a problem, perhaps he is preoccupied with some work or household concern. But do you really think your irritation will help, or make him less forgetful the next time? More likely, it will lead to resentment and sharp words in return. On such occasions, kindness, the open sympathy of the heart, will make your companion feel understood and loved. Certainly you will be happier: not only will you feel the love of your partner for your understanding, but you will be content with yourself for your wisdom. Mutual forgiveness for small failings can be a genuine inspiration for love. You know that I am not encouraging tolerance of serious failings and problems: these should be confronted and resolved. But innocent failings – and who does not have them? – can be the irregular side of a puzzle piece that allows two people to lock together.

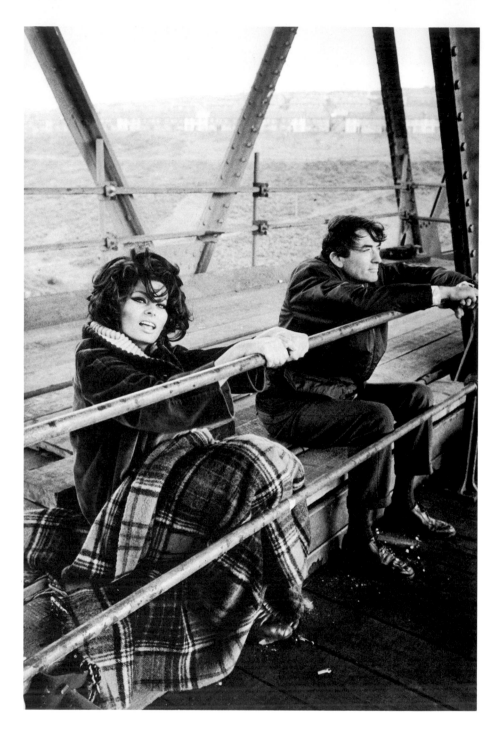

Filming Arabesque *with Gregory Peck, one of the most charming men I have ever met.*

Most examples of kindness are so small that they evaporate in the heat of an examining light. But believe me, these kindnesses amount to love. They are the grains of sand in the cement that binds a couple together.

Freedom Is the Spine of Love

You must be free in your love or it is not real love. We all know and accept this with our minds, but it is not so easy in practice. The more difficult aspect of freedom in love is allowing the other person to have it. I don't mean freedom to do anything according to whim – that would be damaging to the couple's bond. I am talking about allowing your loved one the freedom to be himself.

Here is a scenario we all recognize. Mary and Tom are at a party. Perhaps Tom drinks a bit too much. Mary starts to frown. Tom begins to tell his story of losing his luggage in Guatemala. The frown breaks into a scowl. Mary, grabbing Tom's arm, says that everyone has heard that story. Tom tells the story, oblivious of her irritation. Mary spends the rest of the evening trying to rein him in. When she finally gets Tom alone, she refuses to speak to him and the next morning she is only too pleased that he has a hangover.

Doubtless we have all had occasions when we have winced at our man's behavior. Carlo, for example, tends to fall asleep at parties. But I think we must, difficult though it seems, admit that this person, this husband or lover, is not a part of us. He has a right to his innocent quirks of behavior. Probably no one at my mythical party was bothered by Tom's obvious enjoyment of the evening. Perhaps no one had heard his luggage story. Indeed, if there was any discomfort, it was no doubt caused more by Mary than Tom. Most often in these cases, sympathy is with the renegade spouse.

I use this example of the couple at the party because it is such a common one. But you can think of many situations in which you feel the desire to make your man conform to your standards even in simple ways. We seem to have this drive to make the other person into what we consider a perfect version of himself. It is so curious that we are attracted to people for certain reasons, and then, once we are together, we often try to change those very things that first drew us. Once upon a time, Mary was probably attracted by Tom's spirited ways; now she would prefer that he become reserved, like herself.

The next time your lover does something that you find irritating, stop and think a minute why it upsets you. Is there really anything wrong with what he is doing? If in fact his action is innocent, why not relax and let him be himself? You will both find life easier when, lovingly, you grant each other the freedom to be yourself.

PREGNANCY AND MOTHERHOOD

My first pregnancy was the most extraordinary period of my life. I had wanted a baby for years, had suffered two miscarriages, which had thrown me into despair and, at last, at the age of thirty-four, I had conceived again. Because the doctor I trusted lived in Switzerland, I move to Geneva to be near him. If I had had to move to the North Pole and live in an igloo for nine months to wait for my baby, I wouldn't have hesitated.

Pregnancy should be a magical time for a woman, but for me it was not. I was terrified that I would lose my baby. Confined to a hotel, in bed most of the day, I made every effort to stay calm – which, for me, was almost impossible. My emotions were always at war: yes, I am pregnant and about to become a mother and soon I will hold my little baby and be the happiest woman on earth; no, I must not get my hopes up too high or I will invite a tragedy. I awoke every day relieved to have safely passed another twelve hours, and went to bed at night with the same thought.

It wasn't always so grim. I did have diversions. I became interested in cooking. Fortunately, that is something you can do when you are in a hotel room for nine months! After trying out all the recipes I could remember from my childhood and experimenting with some new ones, I collected them all into a cookbook. In addition to cooking, I read. Not books about babies and baby care – I thought that might be tempting fate. But I read novels and biographies, and read and reread magazines that told me what was going on in the rest of the world. Friends visited me and that was always a great pleasure.

I remember when Vittorio de Sica came to see me. There had been so many rumors about my condition. Of course, the press had reported that I had suffered miscarriages and that I longed to have a child. When I disappeared into a hotel in Geneva, it quickly became known that I was waiting for a baby. But the press invented the story that I had hidden a pregnant woman in the hotel with me and that when she had her child I would say it was my own. It is a credit to the power of the press that so many people believed this – even, as it turned out, my dear friend De Sica, who should have known better. When he came to see me I was seven months pregnant and, as I am not a small woman, when I stood up and threw out my

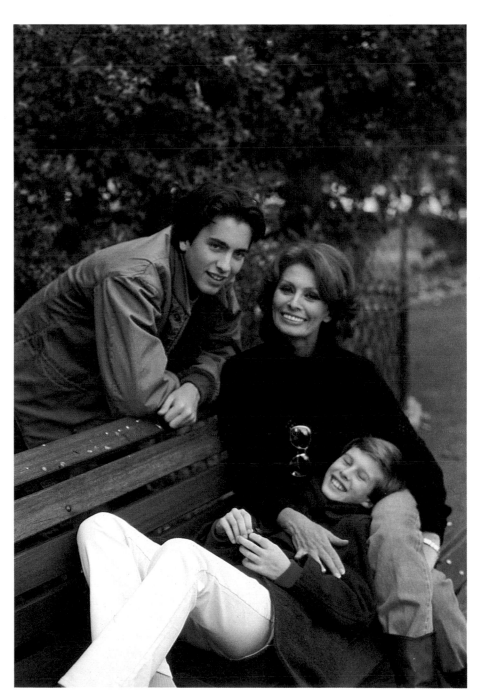

With Carlo Jr and Edoardo in Geneva, 1983.

arms to greet him, I was an eye-filling sight. "Ah," he gasped, "you really *are* pregnant!" The evidence was undeniable.

I should add that these stories in the press never bothered me at all. I was so absorbed by my pregnancy that nothing else could touch me. And I don't blame De Sica for believing them. I have found myself that even when I know for a fact that something I read in the newspapers isn't true, if it is about someone I know, it sticks in my mind. It is a terrible thing and a fact of life for anyone in the public eye.

The experience of pregnancy and motherhood has a strange effect on a woman. In one sense it isolates you from the rest of the world, as it isolated me from those press reports: you are entirely engrossed in your own body and the life it holds. It is as if you were in the grip of a powerful force, as if a wave had lifted you above and beyond everyone else. In this way there is always a part of a pregnant woman that is unreachable and is reserved for the future – her baby. At the same time, when you are pregnant you take on a new role that makes you part of the world as never before. When you are a mother, you are never really alone in your thoughts. You are connected to your child and to all those who touch your lives. Before, you could come and go as you pleased, get angry, be impatient, burn your bridges. But a mother always has to think twice, once for herself and once for her child. She needs the world to be safe and happy.

Your Doctor

When you are pregnant, you are dependent, perhaps for the first time in your adult life. Your rely on your husband to help you in physical ways as your body becomes awkward, and you count on him to help you sustain this family that you are both creating. You may find that you are depending on your relatives – your mother, sister or brother – for support. But sometimes you will get conflicting advice or you will have unique problems, and then your biggest dependence is on your doctor.

A doctor can be the most important figure in a pregnant woman's life. I know that today women are educated about their bodies and eager to make choices concerning their health care. Taking this responsibility is very important. But this approach should not be in conflict with reliance on a doctor. Take the time to find a physician you trust. Make sure his ideas about pregnancy and delivery agree with your own. Some doctors are autocratic about everything from vitamins to drugs during labor, while others adopt a relaxed role. The style of your doctor doesn't matter as long as you are comfortable with it.

My own doctor, Dr. Hubert de Watteville, was a hero to me because he seemed to care as much as I did about my babies. I am very sad as I write

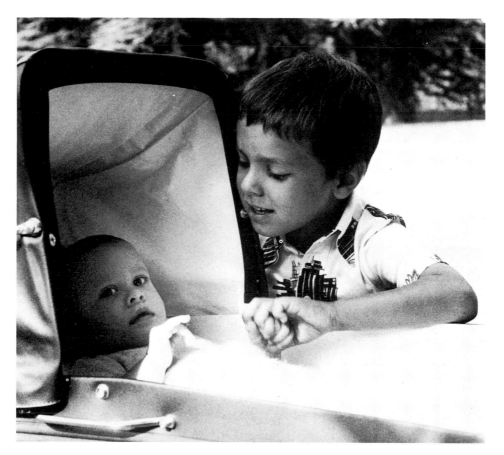

Five-year-old Carlo Jr scrutinizes the new arrival but does not seem too jealous.

this because he recently died and I lost a friend as well as a man who changed my life in the most profound way. My comfort is that a man who brought so much life and happiness into the world will always be alive in some way.

Dr. de Watteville was wonderful to me during my pregnancies and I trusted him completely. He was very relaxed with me, and I realized later that much of what he did was dictated by my great fear of losing my baby. If he had been strict, I would have been even more nervous, and heaven knows what would have happened. For example, he taught me all the natural childbirth breathing exercises, although he told me later that he always knew I would need a cesarean section. He thought that if I knew of the operation in advance I would be frightened, and he also realized that learning the exercises would help me pass the time. He seemed to sense just how much instruction would be comforting and when it would inspire anxiety.

Dr. de Watteville was really more than a doctor to me. He didn't just guide me through my pregnancy, he kept me from losing yet another baby. In the middle of the third month, I began to feel that odd light-headed feeling that I had had when I lost the other two babies. I was terrified, but Dr. de Watteville gave me an injection of an extra dose of estrogen, and within a day I was fine.

Not every woman can have or would need the kind of devoted care I had from Dr. de Watteville, but whatever your circumstances I urge you to find someone, a doctor or midwife, who shares your approach to pregnancy and will make you feel secure and happy at this most important time in your life.

Advice, the Plague of Motherhood

The biggest problem facing a pregnant woman is not nausea or fatigue or her wardrobe – it's free advice. If you have just had your heart broken, you can go to the market and buy groceries in peace. If you have just got a new job, you can tell people in your own way. But if you are pregnant, your body takes over and sooner or later announces the big news in your life. Everyone from the garage mechanic to the childless waitress will have advice for you.

Free advice is a cross that all mothers have to bear almost from the moment they conceive to the end of their lives. It begins in pregnancy when it is most confusing and dismaying because you are new to motherhood. By the time your child reaches the age of five and someone tells you to slap him whenever he cries, you know enough to realize that this person is crazy. When you are pregnant, you are vulnerable, so you must be prepared.

In my pregnancy I was shielded from much of this advice simply because I was staying in a hotel room and alone much of the time. But I had my share of it. Then once my baby was born I was fair game. I remember my mother, for example. When I told her little Carlo cried in the night, she said this was awful, terrible – what could be wrong with the child? Maria's children all slept through the night from the earliest days. How could my dear mother have forgotten that Maria's babies had cried all night? Some people thought my babies should be fed constantly, others believed in a rigid schedule. If I kept baby Carlo out on a summer evening to play on the grass, it was a scandal. How could I expect the child to be normal when he was up all night?

I learned very quickly to agree with everyone. I would smile and say, "Of course. You are so right. What an excellent idea." Then I would go on doing whatever I knew to be right for my baby. Everyone was happy.

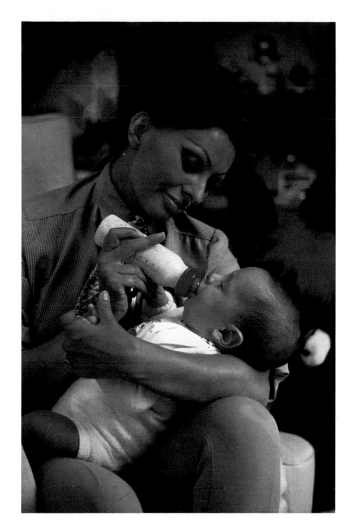

The birth of my first baby was to me the most longed for and joyful event in my life, and I spent all the time I possibly could with him in the early months.

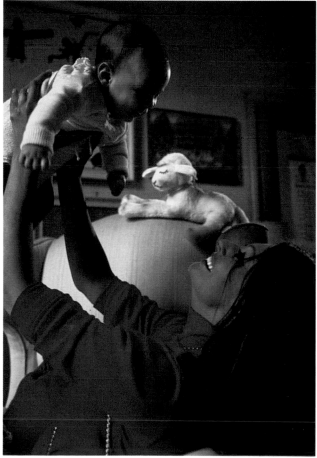

Here is what I finally decided about free advice and I pass it on to you. When you are pregnant, listen only to your doctor. He or she has the latest medical information and, if you have chosen your doctor carefully, will be able to give the right answers to all your questions and allay your fears.

Once your baby is born, follow nothing but your own instinct. Good information is available from many sources and you shouldn't ignore it: a mother has to learn about nutrition and discipline and a host of things that will keep her child healthy and happy. But finally you alone know your child and how to handle him. I think the care of babies would be easier if we could be more relaxed, more confident in our approach and more willing to acknowledge that every baby is different. Carlo was a very fussy baby and I believe that was at least partly because I was an anxious mother. Edoardo was calmer; so was I. Your baby may need to be fed every hour, another baby every three hours. One of the joys of motherhood is learning to know your child so well that you can anticipate his special needs and give him just what he requires to meet the world. Don't let anyone take this privilege away from you.

Beauty in Pregnancy

In my opinion, nothing makes a woman more beautiful than pregnancy because then she is so regal and self-contained. Certainly I have never felt so beautiful as when I was pregnant. In fact, I was never less concerned with my appearance because all I really cared about was having my baby and, for the first time in years, I was alone, unconcerned about photographers, public opinion or how I would look for a particular part. Nonetheless, I spent more time grooming myself than at any other period of my life except perhaps those experimental teenage years. I fussed with my hair, nails, makeup and skin to pass the time. I would wake up, have breakfast, fix my hair, read for a while, give myself a manicure, fuss with makeup, and it would be time for lunch. Half a day was gone and I was that much closer to holding my baby in my arms. I know that if I had had a normal pregnancy I would never have spent so much time on grooming. Still, it is important for a pregnant woman to feel attractive if only to remind herself that she will continue her life as a woman as well as a mother.

To some degree, a pregnant woman must abandon her figure. A trim figure should be your last concern. You must pay attention to good nutrition, but you shouldn't be counting calories and trying to stay slim. In order to be healthy yourself and have a healthy baby, you will gain weight – sometimes quite a lot of weight – and your thighs and arms and face may seem full. This is normal. Once you have your baby, breast-feeding and exercise will help you regain your figure. It may take some time to get back to your original weight – some women find that it takes almost a year. But don't be discouraged. Be patient with your body. I saw a friend a few months after she had a baby and she was so depressed because she hadn't lost all the weight she had gained during pregnancy. I tried to encourage her to relax. It really made me sad to think that some women are so concerned about their figures that a few extra pounds can affect their mood so strongly. I know that it is difficult to lose weight, but once your baby is a few months old and your time is somewhat more your own, you will find that with some real effort the weight will disappear.

A good, balanced diet is important during your pregnancy. Because I am always careful what I eat, I had no special diet: I just ate a bit of everything as always, without gorging, and took a vitamin supplement. For the first four months of my pregnancy, meat revolted me, so I avoided it. The only change in my regular diet came at seven months when Dr. de Watteville told me to cut down on salt, as I was retaining too much water. He said that I couldn't tell because I saw my face every day, but he noticed that I was getting puffy. So I cut down on salt, and that problem was solved.

Exercise, like diet, should be a continuation of your prepregnancy routine, with any modifications your doctor may suggest. If you have never exercised, now is not the time to begin a rigorous program, but if you have always taken a lot of exercise, there is no need to stop suddenly unless there are complications. I didn't exercise at all until the seventh month of my pregnancy, but that was because the doctor was afraid that any exertion might contribute to another miscarriage. Eventually I did simple exercises and walked around the room. It wasn't as nice as my regular walking in the mountains of Switzerland, but at least it got my circulation going. You might find that an exercise class for pregnant women is beneficial, as well as being a good way to meet others who share your interests and concerns.

As your pregnancy progresses, you may begin to feel ungainly and awkward. This is the time when you really need to pamper yourself. Experiment with makeup. Try new products, especially different ones for your eyes, as attractive eyes will always make you look pretty. Don't neglect your hair. Keep it clean and styled, and get it cut as often as necessary. This isn't the time to have it looking ragged. You may have trouble reaching your toes for a pedicure and if so, don't worry about them too much. But give your fingernails special attention: keep your cuticles creamed and the nails trimmed. I tried out new nail polish colors that ordinarily I would never wear, and they made me feel quite glamorous.

Your skin needs extra care when you are pregnant. I used lanolin on my tummy and breasts every day, beginning around the third month, to prevent stretch marks. I never went outside, but I hope you do, and if you are in the sun, use a sunblock on your skin. The hormones of pregnancy make your

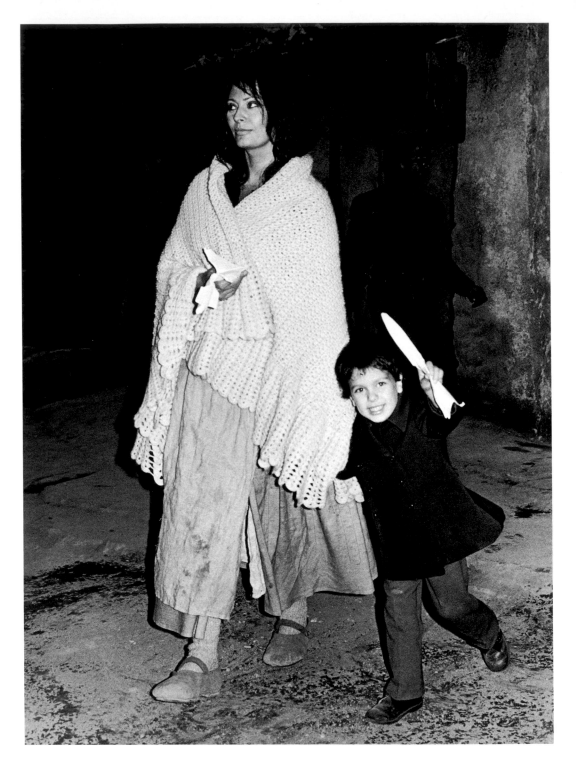

My beloved little Carlo visiting me on the set of Man of La Mancha.
He delighted in my acting disguises, thinking they were just for fun.

skin more vulnerable to being burned. Also you may have moles or slight skin discolorations that will be aggravated by unprotected exposure to the sun. If your skin is dry, be lavish with your use of body creams. Gently massaging creams into your skin can help circulation while it smooths the skin.

Rest and relax whenever you can, for your own health and that of your baby. Take naps. Put your feet up on pillows to prevent varicose veins and swollen ankles. Take baths to relax and soothe you. Just remember when you are pregnant to stick to milk baths; don't use oils or perfumes or bubbling lotions because you might have an allergic reaction to them. And don't let the water get too hot, as that can hurt you and your baby – it should be just slightly above body temperature. When you step out of your bath, while your skin is still damp, rub moisturizing lotion all over. Toward the end of your pregnancy, when you bathe be careful that you don't slip. You might have your husband help you in and out of the tub, and he can also lend a hand by massaging lotion into your skin after the bath.

I think that the role of beauty care during pregnancy is to make you relax, to give you pleasure and to make you feel proud of yourself. Take the opportunity to forget about how others react to you and your appearance and think only of yourself and your baby. Don't abandon your grooming rituals, though; savor them more than ever.

Being a Mother

At the end of my thirtieth week of living in that hotel in Switzerland, my moment had arrived. Dr. de Watteville came in the evening and told me that at six o'clock the next morning, a car would drive right into the ballroom of the hotel to avoid photographers, pick me up and take me to the hospital. My baby would be delivered by cesarean section and it would all be over by lunchtime. It was ending, this pregnancy. I did not sleep at all that night. All I could think of was that I didn't want this child to leave me. I didn't want my pregnancy to end.

I remember every moment of that night and the next morning, every step down the corridor of the hotel, the car ride in the dark morning, the hospital room. I heard a baby cry in the next room and thought how in a few hours I would hear my own baby cry. In those moments I would willingly have waited an eternity to hear that cry. I wasn't frightened. I just didn't want to give up this baby who was so completely mine.

Now I know that this was the first moment of motherhood. This was the beginning of giving up my child to his own life. Pregnancy is one thing; motherhood is another.

As a woman waits for her baby, she becomes more tolerant and courageous. She is trusting. She builds armor against anxieties. When she gives birth, she is unreachable in her loneliness. Her thoughts are on the biological event and all she has is faith. When her baby is born, she needs all the courage and tolerance and trust she has developed. The wisdom that she has gained in the pregnacy and birth may seem like a small thing at first – she may even be unaware of it – but gradually it will give her the strength she needs to be a mother.

You may have guessed by now that I believe that motherhood is the greatest role of my life. Nothing, not even winning an Oscar, can compete with the pleasure and sense of accomplishment it has given me. I believe that all women feel an instinctive urge to make a family. Some women may use this desire creatively in their work or by living lives devoted to ideas. For me, nothing could substitute for motherhood.

When I became pregnant, my concern for my career evaporated. Nothing mattered to me but my baby. If necessary, I would have given up my work to have a child. If this means I am not modern, then I am not modern. I believe that an infant needs to be with its mother as much as possible. This closeness, the endless flow of attention are the accumulation of love that a child carries through his life as a heritage. If you are lucky, your early childhood memories are intense, warm moments of love, of security, of your mother watching you or helping you. It seems to me that people with these happy memories are content as adults because they can still recall the powerful security of being totally loved, while those with memories of being frightened and abandoned find it difficult to find real peace and happiness.

I am aware of the implications of what I am saying and, to be honest, a part of me hopes that it is not true. I know that many women today leave their babies at an early age to go back to work. I truly hope that these children will grow up joyful and that my ideas are outdated. But I wouldn't be honest if I said that I thought a few hours in the evening after a day's work could substitute for day after day spent with your baby.

If you share this desire for children and a yearning to be with them, don't worry about not being modern. Follow your instincts and enjoy your children to the fullest. If you feel secure in your pleasure at being a mother, your children will sense it and life will be easier and happier for the whole family.

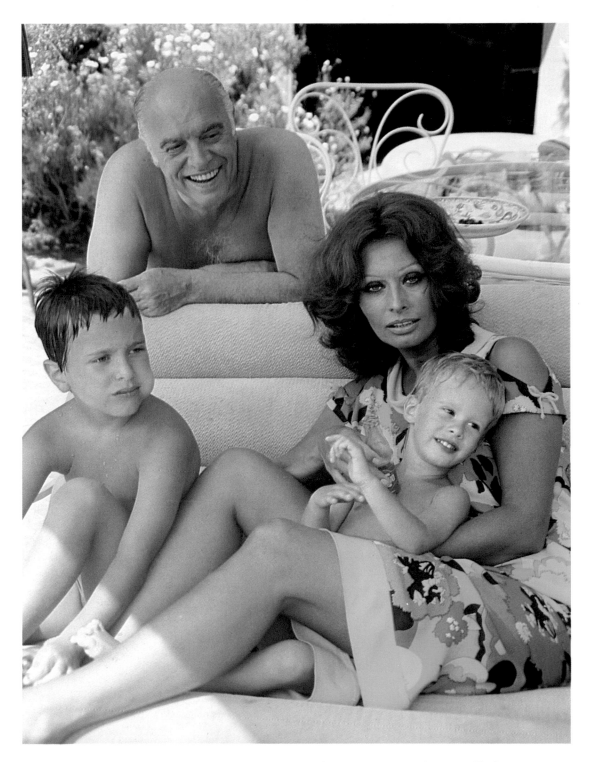

With the two boys and Carlo by the swimming pool at our villa in Marino, near Rome, 1976.

TRANQUILITY

When I began to gather my thoughts about women and beauty, I wanted to say something that went beyond my own personal experience. There must be some general principles of beauty, I thought, that I can pass on to my readers. So I tried to think of women who have been considered beautiful through history. Popular images of beauty change as quickly as the weather. But I wanted to find an example of a beauty who had stood the test of time, someone who was beautiful yesterday, is today and will be tomorrow – a classic beauty of art.

The Mona Lisa of Leonardo da Vinci quickly came to mind. Here was an image of a woman who had captivated man's imagination through the years. It had been a long time since I had seen the painting and, to be honest, my memory of it had faded. I had come to think of the Mona Lisa as a woman whose beauty had suffered the plague of so many of today's beauties: exposure to the point of annihilation.

It was in this skeptical frame of mind that I visited the famous painting in the Louvre. Looking back at me was a woman with cheeks slightly too full, a mouth slightly too thin and a nose much like my own, which is to say a nose that the Mona Lisa might have wished were shorter. Well, I decided, there is nothing in this woman's face that will give me any general principles of beauty. She has nice eyes, but she looks as if she could lose a few pounds, and today she probably wouldn't be able to find work if she depended on her face. But as I continued to look at the painting, I realized that, despite the defects apparent to any critical eye, the Mona Lisa is a woman of undeniable attraction. She seems to be trying to tell you something, some secret that will change your life. What, I wondered, could explain the fascination one feels when confronting her?

I found that the Mona Lisa did just what I asked of her: she became an inspiration to me. Under the spell of that compelling gaze, I decided that the source of her famous smile, and therefore her attraction, is tranquility. This was the general principle of beauty I discovered in the Louvre and it made my trip worth while. The Mona Lisa looks like a woman who owns the most precious knowledge in the world – the knowledge of self. There is no beauty that can compare with the beauty of self-knowledge and the tranquility that comes when you accept yourself as you are.

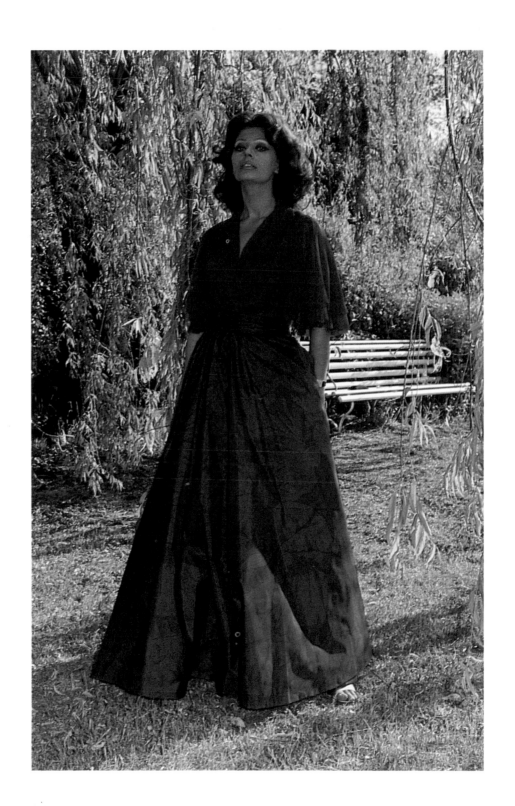

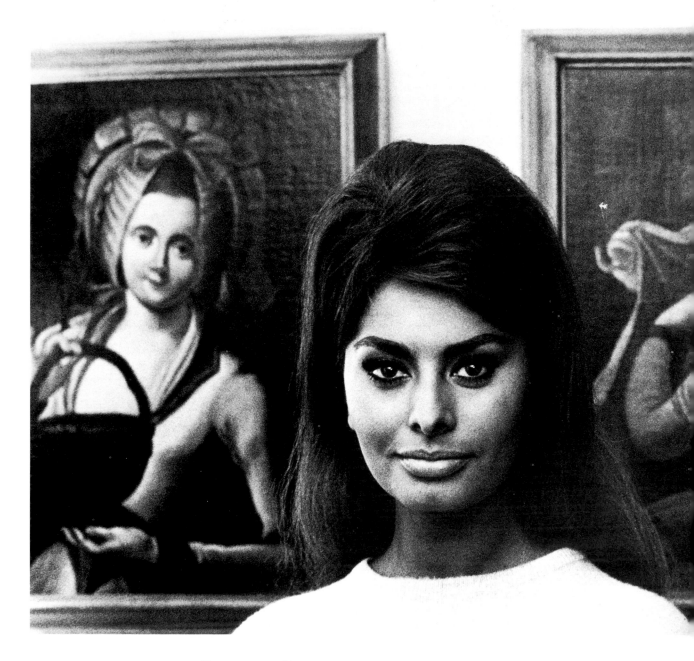

To me, tranquility is a little-sung but vital source of beauty.

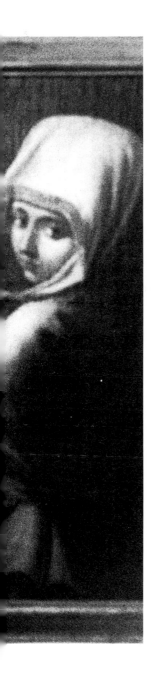

I have already talked about self-confidence as a source of beauty, but there is a difference between self-confidence and tranquility. Self-confidence has to do with the way we face the world, while tranquility reflects the way we face ourselves.

It seems to me that once upon a simpler time it was easier for women to achieve tranquility. This is not to say that a woman's life was carefree in the days before medicine, plumbing, household appliances and all the other conveniences that we now embrace. But in the past a woman didn't choose a life, she accepted one. It is always more difficult to live with a bad choice than a bad obligation. Today you choose your life. You choose if and when and whom you marry. You choose whether or not and when to have children, where to live and whether to work. Even if you don't freely make these decisions for yourself, you are aware that other women are making them and that they are there to be made. Sometimes this awareness makes your own lack of choice in some matter particularly hard to bear. And don't forget that your freedom to choose brings with it the anxiety that is a consequence of freedom.

It isn't easy to make choices in today's complex world. You should recognize the difficulty you face in coping with family and work and obligations to yourself. In order to succeed you must find some sense of balance and certainty that will sustain you. Tranquility is the gift that can help you find real and lasting beauty in your life.

Journalists have often asked me, "What is your biggest beauty secret?" What can I say? I would wonder, struggling to find an honest and believable answer. I usually found a way to divert the conversation, but finally I have discovered that I do have a beauty secret. It is only a "secret" because you never hear or read about it, but I guarantee that it will make you more beautiful. It is a sense of inner peace.

That is really my greatest beauty secret. People have often commented on this quality that I possess, but it is only recently that I have come to appreciate what they mean. I can't take credit for it. If I do have a sense of inner peace, it comes from my history, my experiences, my mother's strength, my personal faith, my children, so many things. And any tranquility that I have is fragile. There are times when I am anything but tranquil. But after the lesson of the Mona Lisa, I have decided that tranquility is a great source of beauty, and so I am more aware of it than ever and I want to share some thoughts with you on this genuine "beauty secret."

Paradoxically, the more you strive for tranquility, the more elusive it becomes. You can't sweat and strain into becoming tranquil, for if you do, you will be like a woman stranded in the desert, finding that the water disappears just as she reaches to cup it to her lips. Tranquility is more a matter of being receptive – receptive to the small pleasures of life and to the

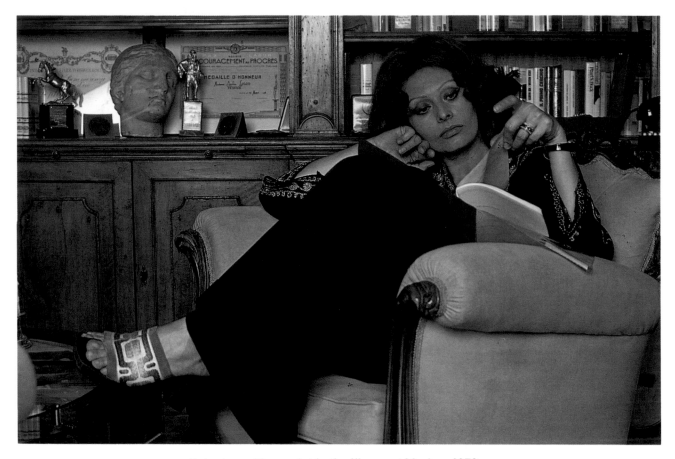

Relaxing with a script in the library at Marino, 1978.

satisfaction of goals achieved. (Aren't you relieved at last to have a beauty secret that doesn't demand constant vigilance?) For me, the pleasure of being with my family, especially my children, gives me the greatest tranquility. Of course, I take pleasure in my work, but not because of the glamor associated with it, rather because it is a goal set and then achieved.

You can't seize upon tranquility any more than you can learn the source of the Mona Lisa's smile. You must be open to it so that it can find you. But there are some techniques, some "devices for the spirit," that can make you more receptive to tranquility.

Organization

Organization. Such a dull word. So full of obligation. Sometimes all I need to do is hear the word "organization" to think how I long to be a blithe spirit living by instinct alone. Most people probably have this response when they know that they are about to be told to become organized. We like to pride ourselves on our spontaneity because the freedom to be disorganized seems to belong to youth. I see it in my sons: I call it the "leg over the arm of the chair" syndrome. Youth is always ready to move at a moment's notice but is generally disinclined to move on anyone else's orders. Well, I propose that we change our minds about organization, that we consider organization as something that will free us, something that will make our lives easier and more pleasurable. Maybe as a bonus we will find that this new freedom makes us youthful in spirit.

Being badly organized, dashing here and there and always running out of time can exhaust anyone and ruin the best disposition and the best intentions. If you want to be tranquil and have a measure of peace in your life, you have to gain control of your daily activities; you must be organized.

It is a mistake to approach organization as a means of grouping disagreeable tasks into one solid stretch of misery followed by a reward of a few pleasurable hours. It is more beneficial to find ways of making your chores a source of satisfaction. This takes some thought and some effort, but in my opinion it is well worth the trouble.

Here is what I mean by organizing for pleasure. We all have certain tasks that we avoid because we don't enjoy them. I find this avoidance is the most disrupting factor in my life. Because I don't want to write a letter or make a telephone call or iron a blouse, I put it off; but it lingers in my mind, haunting me and reminding me of how inefficient and lazy I am. I feel guilty, and no matter what I do, I am robbed of pleasure by the specter of my avoided task.

Now, there are always going to be things that you don't want to do, but think how much more enjoyable your life would be if whenever possible you found a way to incorporate pleasure into your chores. Say, for example, you hate washing the dishes. It is certainly not the most exciting way to spend an hour. Well, try lightening it by adding an element of pleasure. Keep a radio in your kitchen and listen to some favorite music or an interesting discussion while you work. One night when I was living in Paris, I had invited some friends over for dinner. There was no one there to do the dishes, and I hate to walk into a dirty kitchen in the morning, so I invited my guests to keep me company while I washed up. Of course, my ulterior motive was a little extra help, but everyone joined in and the party continued in the kitchen as we laughed and talked and finished up all the wine. It became a special night because everyone was so relaxed and intimate. If I had waited until morning to do the dishes, it would have been a lonely job.

Perhaps you avoid writing letters or even business reports because it is really no fun to sit alone at home and concentrate on your task. And of course there are so many distractions. Why not try gathering your materials and going to the library or some other quiet place where you can sit and work? You will have no other chores claiming your attention, and you will probably find that the change of scenery inspires you. Acomplishing a task in pleasant surroundings can become a double pleasure.

Perhaps you spend too much time on the telephone; when you have a simple message to convey, you get involved in a long conversation. I find that writing a short note instead can save a great deal of time. Get some stationery that you really like, perhaps with your name printed on it. Use a pen with colorful ink. Find some music on the radio. Writing the notes will no longer be an ordeal. (Mentioning the radio reminds me that Carlo Jr. gave me one of those small portable radios with earphones. I wear it all the time when I vacuum. I drive everyone else crazy in the early morning with the noise of the machine while I am having a fine time listening to my favorite tapes!)

The key to organizing for pleasure is to recognize what you don't enjoy and then combine it with something that you do enjoy. That way you are not dividing up your day into black and white, pleasure and pain. Instead, you are improving the texture of your daily life and gaining control of yourself and your time. I cannot promise that this will make you feel youthful, but it will certainly lift your spirits and make you more pleasant to be with.

There is one final aspect of organization that I should mention – the ability to say no. This is one of my biggest faults. Many years ago, Charlie Chaplin told me: "You have one failing you must overcome, Sophia, one thing you must learn if you are to be a completely happy woman. It is perhaps the most important lesson in living – you must learn to say no. You don't know how to say no, Sophia, and that is a serious deficiency."

He was more right than I ever realized at the time. Being able to say no is essential if you want to organize your time and spend your days as you wish. Otherwise you find that you are committed to doing too many things that you don't really care about and sap your energy and spirit. I am afraid of disappointing people, and so I am inclined to say yes to everything. This is really a weakness and I am trying to fight it. I want to be able eventually to say no to things that don't interest me in a graceful and straightforward way. I advise you to make the same effort.

Control

Control is an interesting element of achieving tranquility because usually we think of it in an active sense. We say, "I must get control of this situation. I must take charge." But I believe the greatest peace comes when we recognize the limits of our control. Today women have responsibilities in so many different areas. It seems they are always taking on more. There is nothing wrong with working hard on lots of projects, but at some point you must acknowledge you can't control the outcome of everything you do.

This is one of the first lessons of filmmaking. Collaboration is the rule.

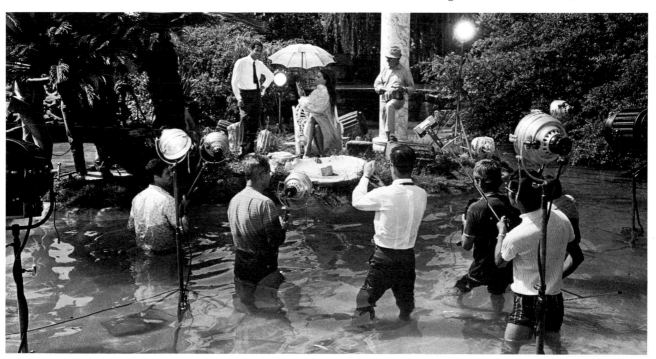

Collaboration was certainly the rule in acquiring the shots for this TV special, taken in the garden at Marino. The result can be seen overleaf.

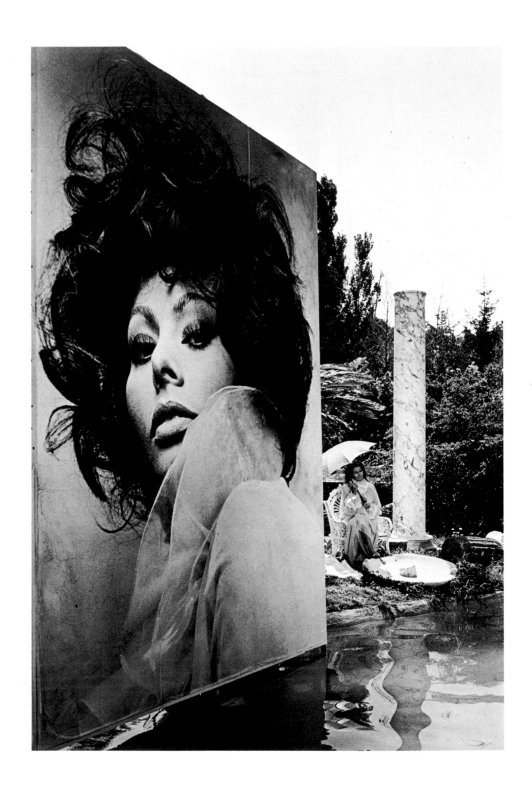

Everyone must bend his efforts toward achieving the best whole. Actors, makeup experts, set designers all find their work to some degree obscured by the art of the film as a whole. Even the director can work only with what is at hand and within the limitations of time, money and weather.

In our lives likewise, we can work only with what is at hand. As daughters, wives, mothers, businesswomen we are beset with limitations. Wisdom comes when you admit your limitations but continue to do your best. The American expression "Take it easy" has a great appeal to me because my impulse is to be impatient. Carlo helped me to learn patience when I began my film career and was eager to get better parts. "Wait five minutes," he would say. It was his version of "Take it easy." Well, now I am much better at taking it easy and waiting five minutes, and this newly learned patience has made a big difference in my life.

My little Edoardo (who is really not so little any longer) taught me a lesson about control when he made a drawing for his older brother, Carlo. As Carlo Jr. was just beginning to play the piano, Edoardo decided to draw the instrument for his brother. What a piano it was! With musical notes flying from its many-colored keys, it amazed me as I watched it take shape. How difficult it was not to correct, not to guide the pencil and explain the black-and-white geometry of the piano that stood a few feet away. I had to curb my impulse to help draw the correct piano. But how limited my vision was compared with Edoardo's! What a delightful instrument he drew, so full of music and joy.

Sometimes it is difficult to stand back and relinquish control. Sometimes the matter is not so simple as a child's drawing. It may be an illness or a husband who works too hard or a misunderstanding with a friend. Still, after you have done all you can, after you have bent every effort, you must recognize that you can't control everything. In some things you are not a director but an actor. When you recognize this, you invite tranquility.

Goals

Nothing brings more joy in life than a goal achieved. Singleness of purpose, wanting to do something and giving it the very best you can – ah, that's what life is all about! Once I am committed to a task, I am fiercely and completely devoted to it, striving for perfection, working as hard and as long as I can to excel. If I hadn't had the talent to be an actress, I would have exploited whatever other gifts I had. I would have been the best teacher in my hometown or the world's best private secretary or a champion sales-woman. Whatever I do, I do with concentration, love and patience, and these forces push me to succeed. This is not braggadocio. It is simply a part of me, like my smile, my walk and my often measured bosom. Nothing has come easily to me. My children, my marriage, my career have all been the result of great struggle. I am on familiar ground when I tell you that hard work and dedication to a goal have brought me greater happiness than anything else in my life.

It is often difficult in the press of daily activities to take the time to survey your life. When you do so, however, you see things in a different and valuable perspective. You have probably heard the expression "An unexamined life is a life not worth living." This is surely true. If you never stop to assess your direction and alter your course, you are probably going nowhere. Just look back on the past year and ask yourself if you accomplished anything that gives you pleasure. Did you learn another language? Have a baby? Learn to knit? Take on a new job? Make a trip that you had longed for? If there is nothing you can see, no partuiclar accomplishment that makes you happy, perhaps you should begin now to think about how you would like to spend this year and the next. The point is not necessarily to make a major accomplishment – although that is always pleasing – but to find goals that are specific and realistic enough to be achieved. Then use your best energies to reach that goal and don't be distracted from it.

I am very lucky because as an actress, for me each film is a new challenge and a new goal. There is a natural rhythm to this that is very gratifying. I am always dissatisfied with my work in my last film and always eager to begin a new one. I hope that when I am ninety, I will still be looking forward to working on new projects.

It is too easy to forget the youthful excitement that comes with working toward an end. Think of a child learning to ride a bicycle. He enjoys such excitement, such a thrill of purpose, such joy when he finally accomplishes his goal. Why deny yourself that same pleasure? If your days are passing without any real sense of anticipation for what tomorrow holds, peace and tranquility will elude you.

Reassessing your goals may force you to decide if you like the direction your life is taking. At times you get set on a course that is good for you, but good only for a limited period of time. Sometimes I think I have spent all of my life being old; that is, being mature and sensible and hardworking. Growing up in poverty and without a father, I was a husband to my mother and a father to my sister; I didn't have the chance to be young, to be frivolous. Perhaps it is time for me to think about being a girl for the first time. Although I don't know whether I could, I mention it because it might help you to think about your life from a fresh perspective.

It is important today for every woman to have something in her life beyond marriage. If I had my life to live over again, I don't think I would be as eager to be married so young. Of course, when I was a girl, marriage was the

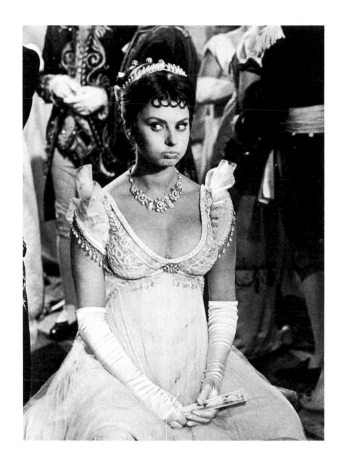

Each character and each film presents a fresh challenge and demands something new from me. Here I can be seen as a pouting princess in Madame Sans-Gêne, *and dressed as a nun for a film of Luchino Visconti's which sadly was never made.*

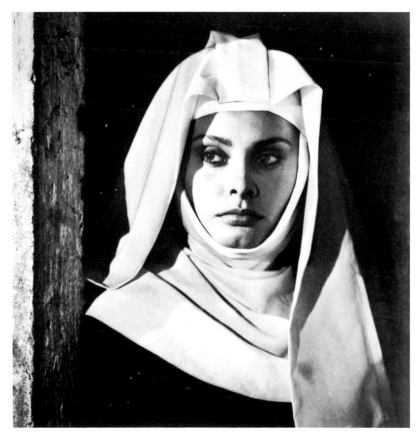

main goal for a woman; anything else was just a bonus. But I have come to think that it is important for a woman to have something more in her life that is hers alone. Otherwise, when the children leave home, what is she to do with herself? This is a problem that many women face today. I am very proud of my sister Maria, who recently got her doctorate after four years of study. I think it must be very difficult to sustain yourself over such a long course of study when there are so many discouragements and distractions. But Maria and many other women these days are doing just that – sustaining themselves and their children with their determination.

Sleep

Recently I had a laugh when I looked through some old clippings of interviews I have given through the years. It seemed that I was always singing the praises of a good night's sleep. Well, in fact, I still think that sleep is an often-overlooked source of tranquility. This isn't just because of the obvious fact that when you sleep you are not worrying about your problems, for I believe that while you are asleep you are often unconsciously working them out. In any case, to me, sleep is very important and can never be considered a waste of time.

Many people don't get nearly enough sleep. We all know those who take a certain pride in saying that they only need four or five hours of sleep a night. Perhaps for some people this is all right. But I don't think it is good for most of us. For me nine or ten hours of sleep are necessary if I am to have a successful day. The quality of my day depends on the quality of my night.

I am not the only one in my family who believes in the restorative power of sleep. Once at a Cannes film festival that he might prefer to forget, Carlo was a member of the jury judging the films. At one morning screening, the first film shown was Truffaut's *The Four Hundred Blows,* and Carlo was there in the front row despite a very late party the previous night. Well, the newspapers next day featured a photograph of Carlo, sound asleep in his seat, with the caption "Not even Truffaut's *Four Hundred Blows* could wake Carlo Ponti!"

If your sleep is to be beneficial, it is important to set your mind on positive thoughts before you fall asleep. Don't think about your problems. If you have trouble putting your mind at rest, try reading. I keep a book beside my bed and read a bit every night to bring my thoughts into a world of fantasy and imagination. Of course, you have to choose your book carefully – the night I started to read Umberto Eco's *The Name of the Rose* I became so engrossed in the story that I stayed up half the night.

If you have trouble sleeping, you should try to set up regular sleep habits.

Go to bed every night at the same time so your body knows when to expect to sleep. Take a brief, warm (never hot) bath to relax yourself. Drink a glass of milk; the calcium in milk really does act as a sedative. Or you might take one or two calcium tablets, as these also encourage sleep. Don't do any vigorous exercise before bed because it will stimulate you and make it more difficult to fall asleep. I have a friend who uses what she calls a "sleep pillow" that she made herself. It is just a square of silk (although you can use cotton) filled with dried rose petals, orange rind, powdered cloves, and some herbs like rosemary, thyme and lavender. She tucks it into her regular pillow and says that the scent helps her drift off to a peaceful sleep. And last but certainly not least, making love is a marvelous soporific.

Solitude

If you wish to invite tranquility, I think you must learn to enjoy solitude. Solitude that is chosen and not enforced is a true plasure. When you are alone, your thoughts can move freely and without interruption. You can find solutions to things that have been troubling you.

I discovered early in life that I am my own best company, and I relish solitude as a means of regenerating myself, especially if I have problems or feel sad. I don't have to have a problem to long for solitude, however. I take pleasure in time spent on my own just walking, reading, listening to music or even doing small chores that have piled up. Sometimes I pick up a dustrag and wander around my apartment cleaning and humming to myself. I know the maid may occasionally think that I am trying to prod her to greater efforts, but I am really just losing myself in a routine task. It is like active meditation for me. In a hectic day, being by oneself just for a few minutes can be a small island of peace. Even when others are at home with me, I sometimes need to be alone. I lock myself in the bathroom for a few minutes at a time and let my mind wander and refresh my spirit.

Sometimes a day or a weekend spent alone, or largely alone, can be the equivalent of spending time at a spa. It can make you hear your own rhythms that are drowned out in the noise of a busy life. What a pleasure it is to take a trip, perhaps to visit a good friend in another city, by yourself. Or even to go to a museum for the afternoon without anyone to distract you in any way. Many women find that a morning spent wandering alone from store to store, looking and shopping, can completely restore their spirits, and I can certainly understand it. Though shopping doesn't intrigue me, I do a lot of traveling and sometimes I relish the thought of getting on a plane where I can be all alone with no obligations for a few hours. I have done some very profitable thinking on plane journeys.

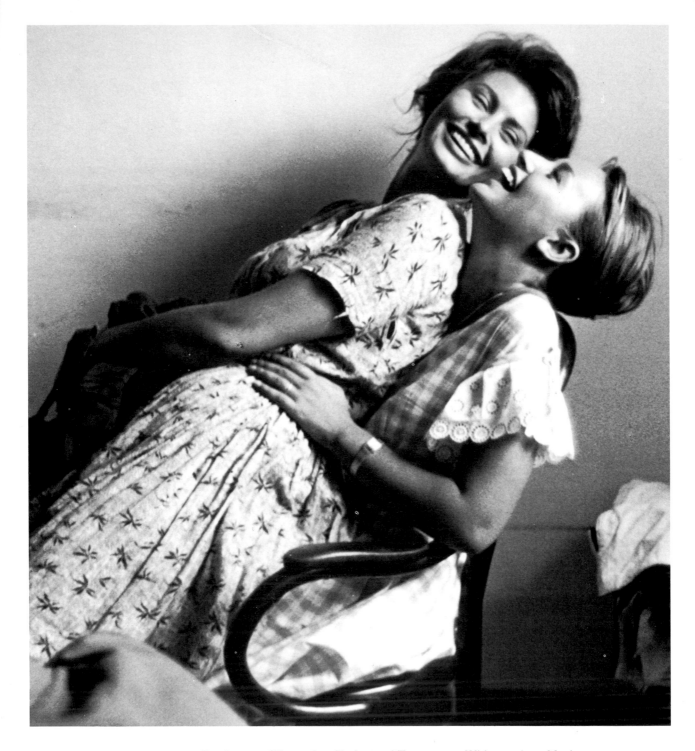

On the set of Yesterday, Today and Tomorrow. *With my sister Maria
I am always happy and relaxed.*

Friendship

Thinking about travel and shopping brings friendship to mind. As I have said, I am not so fond of shopping, but the few times that I do shop I am usually with a friend and we always have fun. It can be a brief holiday, a sort of adventure, to go into a store together and look at things and compare tastes and, of course, laugh. Women are very lucky to have so many opportunities in their lives for friendship.

When I think of friendship, naturally I include my friends. I have only two or three close friends, but they are so valuable. I don't believe you can have lots and lots of friends; you simply can't keep up with more than a few people in a satisfying and intimate way.

A true friend is a rare find. Such a person allows you to be truly yourself, for honesty is at the heart of friendship. Of course, you can only be honest with someone you trust and who cares about your welfare. It takes time to develop a friend. Once you have someone with whom you can share your life, you are lucky indeed.

Naturally every friendship is not a lasting one. People come and go throughout your lifetime, and sometimes the course of a friendship is brief. One of my regrets as an actress is working very closely with people on a film and then having to say good-bye to them. You know that even if you keep in touch, you will never have the same intense friendship that you shared when you were working together. I treasure so many moments of these special friendships. For example, Anne Kramer (wife of Stanley Kramer) spent hours with me during the filming of *The Pride and the Passion.* It was my first film in English and I barely knew the language. I was terrified that I would make a fool of myself because I didn't even know enough to ad-lib if I forgot a word. Anne helped me memorize my lines every night, and she gave me a book of poems by T. S. Eliot, listened to me read them, and corrected my pronunciation. I will never forget her kindness.

Sometimes, not often alas, you meet a person and you know right away that you will become friends. It is something you feel deeply inside yourself, something you can't explain. Such was the case with my friendship with Ann Strasberg. I met her in 1970 while working with her husband, the unforgettable Lee, on the set of *Cassandra Crossing.* Immediately I fell in love with both of them and their wonderful children. I was very upset when Lee died, and after this tragedy my ties with Ann and her family became stronger. I admire her as a woman of great courage, talent and style. She has made a point in her life of continuing her husband's work, keeping alive the famous Actors' Studio.

Naturally I haven't lost touch with all my co-workers. Basilio Franchina, the executive producer of *Woman of the River* which we made in 1954, became one of my dearest friends. Basilio is an Aquarian, and I believe this astrological sign makes for an excellent friend. He is a sort of conscience to the world and never lets me get away with anything. He is also a philosopher and when you meet a philosopher with a conscience, you know you have some explaining to do. Fortunately, Basilio is not perfect. He can be a terrible fussbudget. When I first called him that, he thought it was a compliment, but then an American friend told him what the word meant. It's a shame because I was so enjoying playing a linguistic joke on someone who has been beating me at Scrabble for twenty-five years!

One of the values of friendships is that they can take pressure off any love relationship in your life. Does this sound odd? I think it is true. You probably expect a great deal of the man in your life: usually, unrealistically, you want him to be the sun and the moon for you. You feel that he ought to understand your every problem and be sympathetic to your every mood. Well, as we all know or will learn, this is impossible. No single person can completely fill your life; you will have thoughts and feelings that he can't understand. This is where having a friend can work magic. There have been times when a conversation with a friend has been just the help I needed, just the understanding that I was missing, to bring me back to my senses. I have never found any solace in professional therapy, but on more than one occasion a good friend has helped me out of my troubles.

Most often when you think of friendship, you think about conversation – the sharing of thoughts and problems and experiences. Sometimes, however, friendship demands silence. Vittorio de Sica, who was one of my closest friends, learned that he was very sick before filming *The Voyage*. By the time we started work on the movie, he and everyone else said that he was better, but I don't know if he really believed it. In this film I play a woman who is doomed to die. Her brother-in-law, played by Richard Burton, takes her on a journey, trying to find a cure for her illness. They fall in love, and the last days of her life are a wonderful awakening to romance and the pleasures of life. *The Voyage* was De Sica's last film, and although I had premonitions during the filming that all was not well, I kept my thoughts to myself. I listened in silence to his direction on how to play a woman who was dying just when her life was suddenly becoming full and happy, and I did the best I could. The last time I ever saw Vittorio was when my work was finished, and after embracing him, I left as he laughed with the girls on the set. A few months later he was dead.

Variety is part of the value of friendship: each relationship is different. You might find that with one friend you are always talking about your husband, with another you can share problems in your work, while another is the perfect companion for travel. Don't expect everything from a friend or you will put unfair pressure on the friendship. It is selfish to be too idealistic

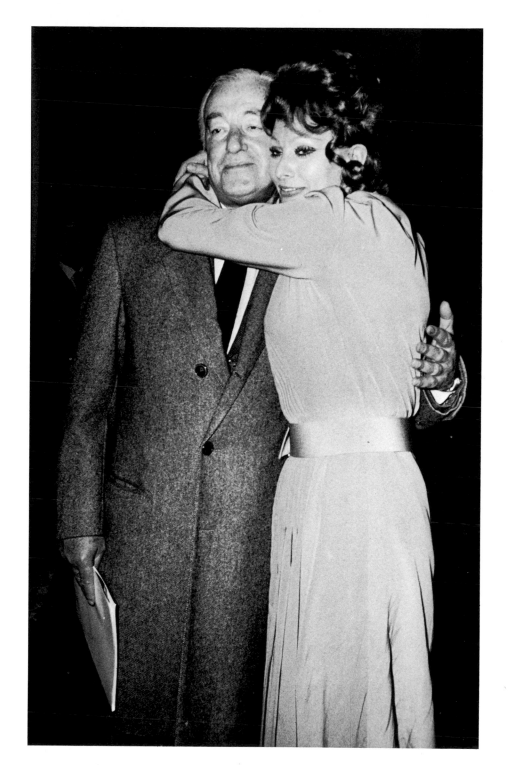

With my unforgettable friend Vittorio de Sica.

about friendship. Find the special qualities of each friend and be grateful for them.

Finally, don't take your friends for granted. Let them know you appreciate them. It is worth nurturing your friendships, for your life would be less rich without them.

Faith

It is easy to lose touch with the spiritual side of one's nature, and this is sad because it can be a great source of peace and tranquility. I have always believed in the existence of a supernatural power. For me, prayer is the link to this spiritual force. But I no longer use the formal prayers that I learned as a child. My prayers are to a God who dwells within me. I am not speaking to heaven when I pray, but to a personal spirit who guides me in my life.

It is unfortunate that today so many people are ambivalent about having faith. The ones who talk a great deal about religion are often extremists, and this must be confusing for young people who are searching for a spiritual identity. I remember one evening in Madrid during the filming of *The Fall of the Roman Empire,* I was walking along a street when I saw Alec Guinness, who was a convert to Catholicism, coming out of a church. He pretended not to see me. I think he was embarrassed to be found leaving a church because he thought I would find it odd. On the contrary, I was impressed by his faith and I thought more of him for having a personal belief.

I don't rely on God to rescue me from trouble or perform any other miracles. Instead, I search for strength to believe in myself and in the people around me. There is no doubt in my mind that if you have great belief you can work your own miracles.

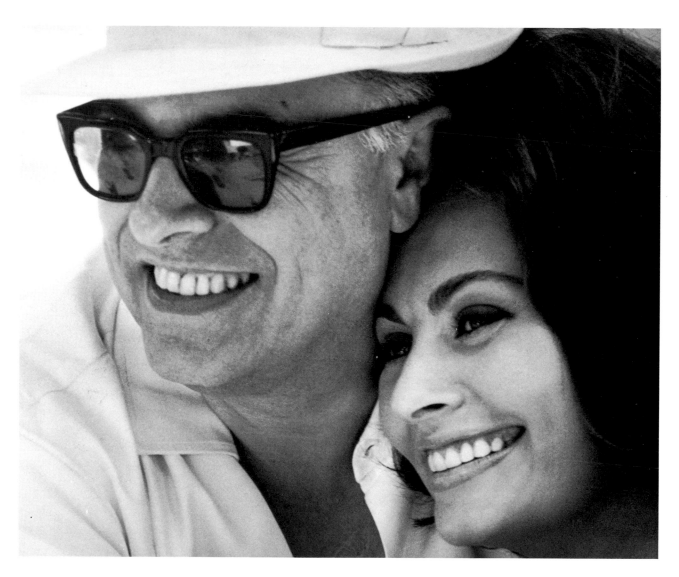

With Carlo, 1968.

COMING TO TERMS WITH AGE

n a magazine article written ten years ago, I said that even though I was about to be forty years old, I felt as if there was some mistake. It seemed that becoming forty was something that happened to other people. Well, now I am fifty, and I have to confess it surprises me every bit as much as it did to reach forty. It is not that I am afraid of being fifty or don't want to be fifty, it is just that the idea of reaching such an age seems incredible to me.

But I am not the same woman that I was at forty, and for that I am glad. Every year has been precious to me despite the difficulties I have faced. I no longer worry about age the way I used to, and I can thank my children for that. Because of them I am always looking forward, anticipating the future rather than longing for the past. Having children keeps you young, because through them you are always learning new things and revising your thoughts and opinions. The very presence of children insists on your future.

As far as my work is concerned, growing older has, I hope, given me greater skill and maturity. I am grateful for the fact that when I started working my aim was to be a serious actress, not a sex symbol whose career was limited by a youthful beauty. I made this choice for practical reasons – I had to support myself and my family – but today I am glad that my career does not depend on having the face of a twenty-year-old. There are actresses who have disappeared entirely because they never developed any real character on the screen, and once the years passed, they had nothing to offer. Of course, this fate awaits any woman, no matter what her work, who has depended on her youthful looks to carry her along.

For me, and I think for many women, thirty was the most difficult birthday. At this age your youth is definitely behind you. You may do wonderful things, but no one will ever again say of you, "Yes, and she's so young too!" You have to begin to take responsibility as an adult. You also have to look at your personal life and see if the direction you are moving in is the right one. For me, the fact that I didn't have children when I was thirty was especially hard to bear. This was so important to me and so crucial for my happiness, but it seemed to be out of my reach, perhaps forever. Fortunately, I was wrong. But at thirty you begin to realize that fresh beginnings are not always awaiting you. The past is with you to stay, for better or worse.

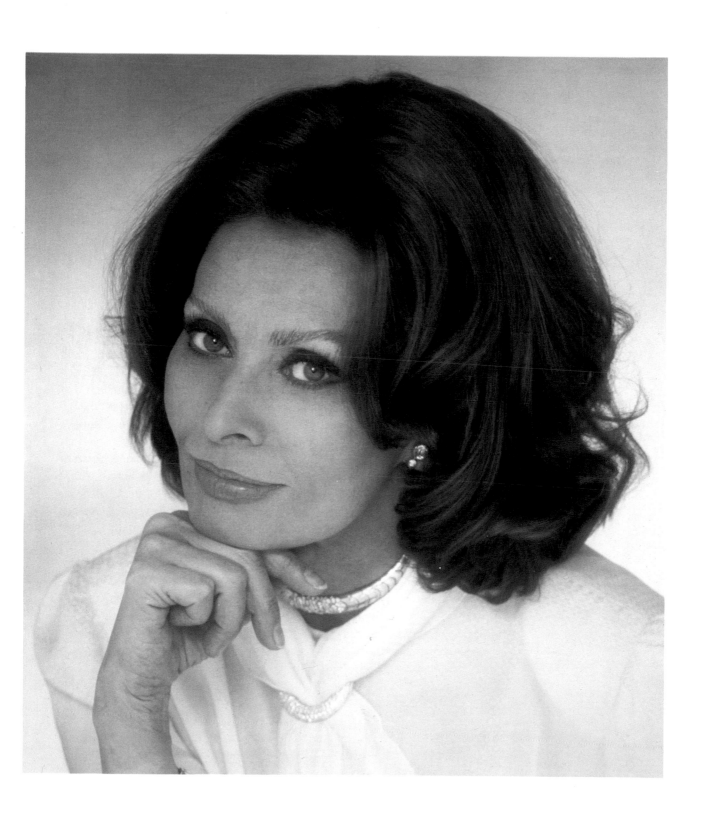

I enjoy being fifty. And if that sounds as if I am just putting a good face on things, I am not. It is the truth. I am so much more comfortable with myself than I have ever been. I know myself much better and I know how to use my time, how to expend my energies and what gives me pleasure. There is an enormous satisfaction in this, and it can only be learned with time.

I have noticed over the past few years that there has been a change in the way the world looks at youth. Remember the "Youth Cult" of the sixties, when anything a young person said had great authority and anyone older than thirty was considered completely out of touch? Today things are different. Life is more difficult for young people, and they are not so confident about the future. They are no longer objects of worship. Now the so-called generation gap has narrowed, and young and old can share their thoughts and feelings. This is good for everyone. It is good for the young because they have a more balanced vision of the world, and it is good for older people because they can take some pride in their experience.

Having pride in your experience will keep you satisfied with your age, whatever it is. If you can look at yourself and know that you have faced difficulties and overcome them, taken risks and dealt with the consequences, gambled with your time and your love and at least sometimes won, then you will feel glad to be the age you are. If, on the other hand, you are not content with your life, if you feel that you have wasted time, have not accomplished the things you dreamed of, not taken chances, not grabbed opportunity, you will wish for the past and regret your years.

The face of a woman tells the world how she feels about her age. You can see it in the face of a woman over forty when she notices a beautiful young girl. If a woman is discontented with her life it will be hard for her to disguise her envy of youth. But if she herself is satisfied, she will watch a young girl with fondness and indulgence.

I am lucky because I have an older woman to look to for inspiration: my mother, Romilda. My mother at seventy-three is still a beautiful woman. She has been beautiful throughout her life, and it has always made me feel more secure about my own future to see how attractive and confident it is possible to be even when you are no longer a girl. I think if there were more women like my mother in the world, we would all feel a little more relaxed about the passing years because we could feel that we have something to look forward to with pleasure.

A Taste of the Future

Most of us spend very little time thinking about what we will look like as we get older. Perhaps we steal a glance at our mothers or grandmothers and wonder, or we see an attractive older woman and tell ourselves that if we

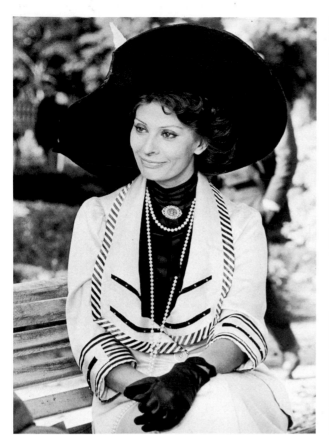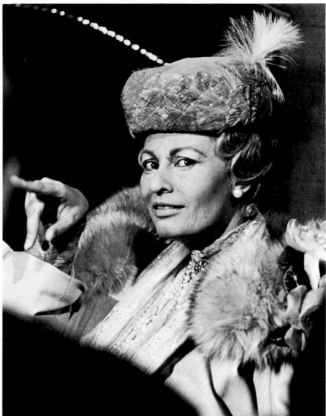

In Lady L *I had the fascinating experience of seeing myself become an old woman.*

could look like her at that age, we would be content. But for the most part the future of our faces is a mystery to us.

I was very fortunate to have that mystery revealed to me when I made the movie *Lady L,* which was released in 1965. In the course of this film, I had to age to eighty years. Before we filmed the final scenes, the makeup artists worked on me, adding wrinkles and thickened skin. It was quite an experience to see my youth disappear before my eyes. And it wasn't just my face that changed; I had to simulate the mannerisms and movements of an old woman. I stiffened my body and hunched my shoulders a bit and squinted my eyes. I not only looked old, I truly began to feel old. But I was pleased to discover that this taste of age was not at all bitter. I looked at this old woman in the mirror and realized that if at that age I was surrounded by my husband, my sons and their wives, and my grandchildren, I would find myself in comfortable terrain.

The experience of becoming an old woman was perhaps more valuable to me personally than any other film experience. I think what we really fear about age is the unknown. We are afraid we will become a different person, less attractive and less valuable. But when you have tried on your old age,

209

you find that it is not so terrible. You are the same person you have always been. It's reassuring.

Mature Beauty

When it comes to appreciating a mature woman's beauty, France is the model country. The French have a history of prizing the appeal of women "of a certain age" – indeed, there is a general feeling that a woman younger than thirty is untried and unseasoned and not as alluring as her older sister. A Frenchman once told me something that I have never forgotten: "Between the ages of thirty-five and forty-five, women are old. Then after the age of forty-five, the devil takes over some women, and they become beautiful, warm, splendid. The acidities are gone and in their place reigns calm. Such women are worth searching for because the men who find them never grow old." Doesn't that make you want to move to Paris? Even if your can't do that you can learn some ways to become "warm and splendid."

The first task women have in creating an enduring image of beauty is to find a completely individual look. Certain women, Greta Garbo or Katharine Hepburn, for example, have highly personal looks and they wear their age with grace. They have discovered what suits them in the way of clothing and makeup, and have stuck with this look throughout a lifetime. In the chapters on elegance and fashion I have discussed ways of finding your special signature. It is not easy, and it takes time and effort, but I believe it is the single most important factor in keeping a woman beautiful throughout her life.

If a woman doesn't have her own look, she is liable to make one of two mistakes as she matures: either she will be a victim of current fashions or she will continue to wear the styles of her youth.

A mature woman who wears whatever is currently fashionable will often look ridiculous unless she chooses with great care and selects only what truly flatters her or is classic in style. Much of what passes for fashion is really a fad. Styles such as midcalf pants, leather bomber jackets, off-the-shoulder sweatshirts and the like are fine for young girls, but on a woman of mature years they create a grotesque contrast between the woman herself and her attemps to look young. Nothing makes a woman look older than an exaggerated effort to look young. Women dressed in youthful fashions resemble little girls putting on their mothers' dresses, high heels and makeup; in both cases, the costume serves only to emphasize their real age.

The other mistake women make, that of dressing in the fashions of their youth, also accentuates age for obvious reasons. If a woman wears what was fashionable twenty years ago (unless what she is wearing is classic), she

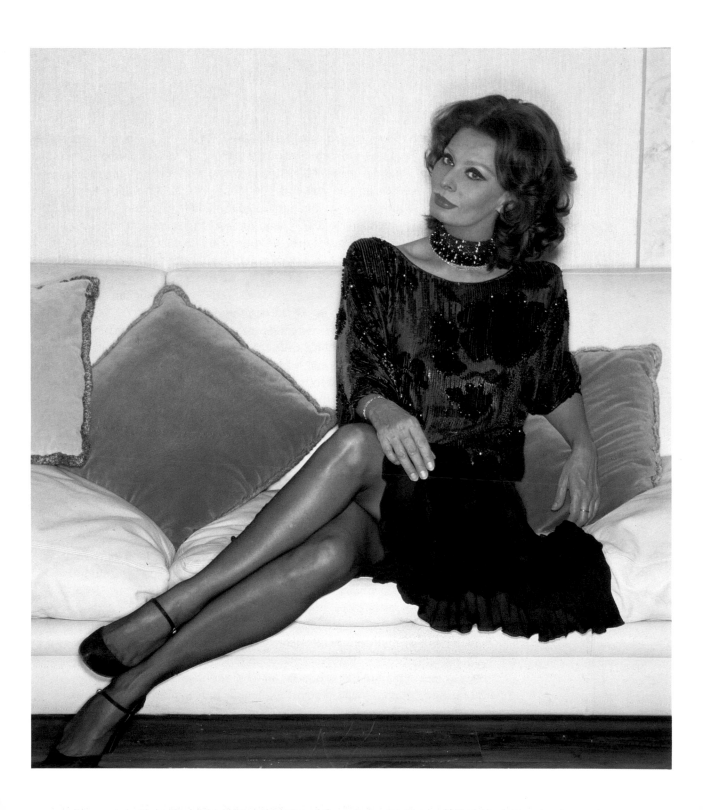

will seem lost in the past and, indeed, older than she is.

As you grow older, you should wear less makeup. This is a simple rule. One often sees older women trying to compensate for their age by wearing more and more makeup, but this is in fact counterproductive. Make sure you use a light touch and also that your foundation is the right shade, for as you age, your skin often becomes lighter in color. You may find that you need little or no foundation most of the time, just cheek color and lipstick, but if you do want to use some foundation, use a very light-textured one – the water-based varieties are the lightest. A good trick, which I have said earlier, is to add a bit of moisturizer to the foundation and mix it in the palm of your hand. This will lighten the foundation and keep your skin moist at the same time. Avoid heavy powder because it will cake and crack. Mascara is important, I think, but false eyelashes look very harsh on an older woman. Keep your eyeliner soft, too: stick to a muted shade and smudge the line.

Cosmetic Surgery

No, I haven't had a face lift. But if the time comes when I feel I want one and I am convinced that it is the right thing to do, nothing will stop me. Even though I feel there is great beauty in the mature woman – and I really believe it – I still think that anything that makes a woman feel better about herself and the way she looks is worth doing.

There are dangers in cosmetic surgery, however, and you must consider it only with your eyes wide open. In the first place, you risk losing your own special look. There is a genius in nature that makes irregularities work together on a face. Sometimes if a nose is shortened or an eye lifted, the face loses its special strength and beauty. I recently read a letter in a magazine from a woman who had had her nose shortened in which she said that this was the worst decision she had ever made in her life. She looked like a different person and she no longer felt like herself. I find the thought of that happening to me terrifying. If you consider cosmetic surgery, you must be confident that you will like the look of the person you will become.

Another and even more important point to think about if you are considering cosmetic surgery is that it is a serious operation. These procedures have innocent names like "tucks," "bobs" and "lifts," but they really are surgery and must not be taken lightly. You can suffer infections, the surgeon can make a mistake, you can have a reaction to the anesthetic – any of the problems you can encounter when you go to a hospital for routine surgery.

If you are still determined to have cosmetic surgery, I think it is essential to see several doctors and compare their methods. Ask to see pictures of women they have worked on. Observe how long the doctors take with you, how they examine your face. I have heard that sometimes a doctor will tell a woman that she shouldn't have anything done to her face. If a doctor tells you this, you should believe it. If another doctor tells you something else, you should have lots of questions for him.

Work and Age

One interesting thing I have discovered as I mature is that in some ways work has become more difficult for me. When I was young, I found myself in the most dramatic and overwhelming situations – starring in a film with Cary Grant, meeting the Queen of England, winning an Oscar. How did I handle all that? Now I realize I was much like infants who are thrown into a swimming pool. Everything was so new and exciting to me and I was unaware of so many things. Like those water babies, ignorance was my best friend. I didn't know enough to be frightened. I just did the best I could, and if I did not fall over or drop food in my lap, I felt satisfied.

Those days of blissful ignorance are gone. People have expectations of me now. I can no longer live by my nerves and rely on instinct. People say, "Let's see how Sophia performs; let's see if she's as good as she's supposed to be." There is less surprise and congratulation if I do well, and less understanding if I don't.

I think this is true for many working people at a certain stage in life. If you have taken risks and have been successful, people now look to you for endurance. You must continue your good work, knowing that people are quicker to see your mistakes and slower to forgive you for them. This realization, that you are being judged more sternly, can be paralyzing if you don't teach yourself to overcome it.

Fortunately, with experience, you will make fewer mistakes. The confidence of accomplishment is there when you need it. I know now that certain roles are all wrong for me, even if the director is good and the film exciting. There is no sense in trying them because they will end in failure. I suppose this is how nature compensates us for losing the nerve of youth: we gain the experience to make better choices for ourselves.

But life would be dull indeed if we simply worked at avoiding mistakes. We must force ourselves to learn, to acquaint ourselves with the thrill of a new challenge by trying something completely different. And sometimes we must do it just for ourselves, without regard for how people around us will react.

There is another benefit to taking chances as you become experienced: you will come face to face with the possibility of failure. After all, experience teaches us that there is a risk in every new endeavor. This is why as we mature we sometimes become reluctant to risk our reputations on

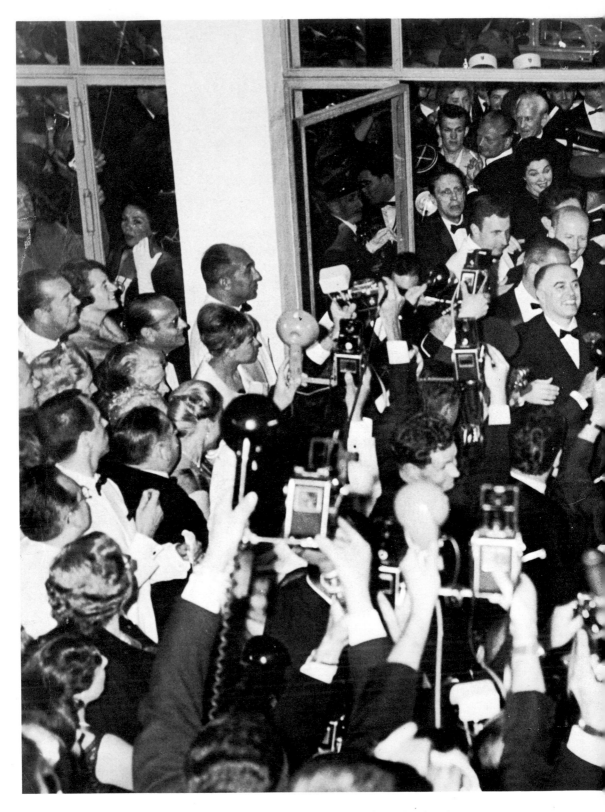

Mobbed by photographers and well-wishers after winning the Palme d'Or at the Cannes film festival for my performance in Two Women *(1961). I was happy, of course, to win the award, but you can see I was also scared.*

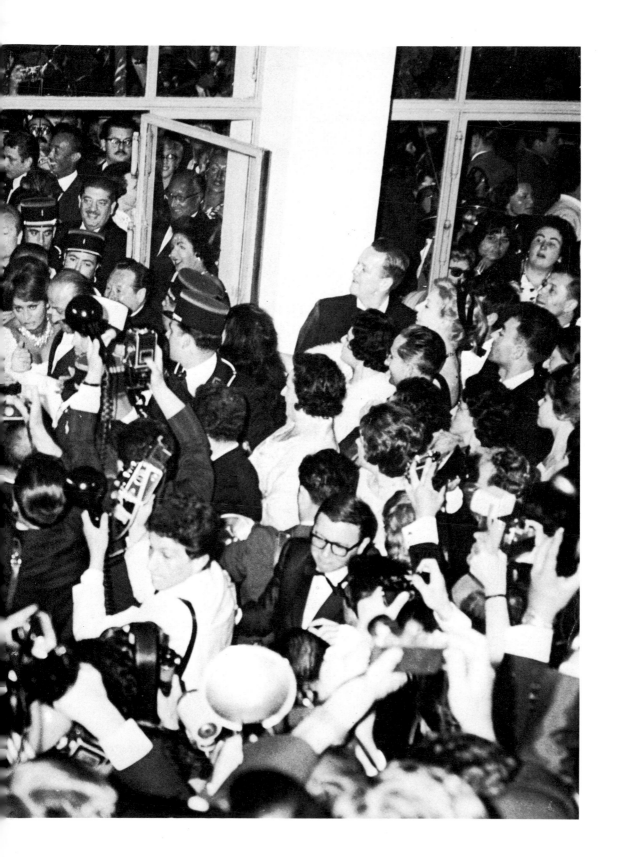

something new. But if you try something and fail, you will have learned a very valuable lesson: failure isn't so awful after all. When you are young, failure teaches you what to avoid, but when you are older, the lesson of failure is different. It is almost relaxing because, much to your surprise, you find that the sun still comes up and you are still hungry for breakfast. And long before you would have imagined, everyone has forgotten all about it. Most people, after all, are much more interested in their own lives than in your mistakes. It is good sometimes to be reminded that life isn't as hard as you had imagined.

There is one last recommendation I want to make about work that perhaps you can apply to your own life. You will be happier and probably more successful if you manage to surround yourself with people you like. Of course you will have to deal at times with people you find abrasive and troublesome. But every time you have a choice in the matter, try to fill your life with people you admire and find agreeable. When I have to deal with people who are aggressive, I am very unhappy. It makes me tense and I behave like an animal cornered in a cage. I am suspicious and guarded. On the other hand, when I am working with people I like, I always do my best. I feel their unspoken support and goodwill, and it truly makes a difference. Working with De Sica and Chaplin, for example, was like performing for best friends. I was able to dare things that I wouldn't have had the courage to try with less sympathetic direction.

It goes without saying that as you grow older, time becomes more precious. Why waste it doing things you don't like, or with people who don't give you pleasure? If nothing else, your experience should have taught you that.

The Fountain of Youth

As we grow older, our bodies begin to fail us in small ways. This is nothing to be frightened of, but it would be foolish to deny the facts. You can no longer stay up very late and arise with a fresh face. You have to work a little harder to keep your figure in shape. Perhaps, like me, you begin to wear glasses to help you read or see from a distance. We are all aware of these subtle alterations – after all, we begin to notice them by the end of our twenties – and we should make efforts to compensate for them. I watch my diet carefully. I am always make sure to use lots of moisturizer on my skin. I am very determined to get enough sleep.

There is one area that many of us don't think about enough, and this is a shame because it should be the first focus of the mature woman. In my opinion, a paradox of aging is that at a time when we find ourselves less confident of our bodies, we often also abandon the one process that is more open to us than ever – the growth of our minds.

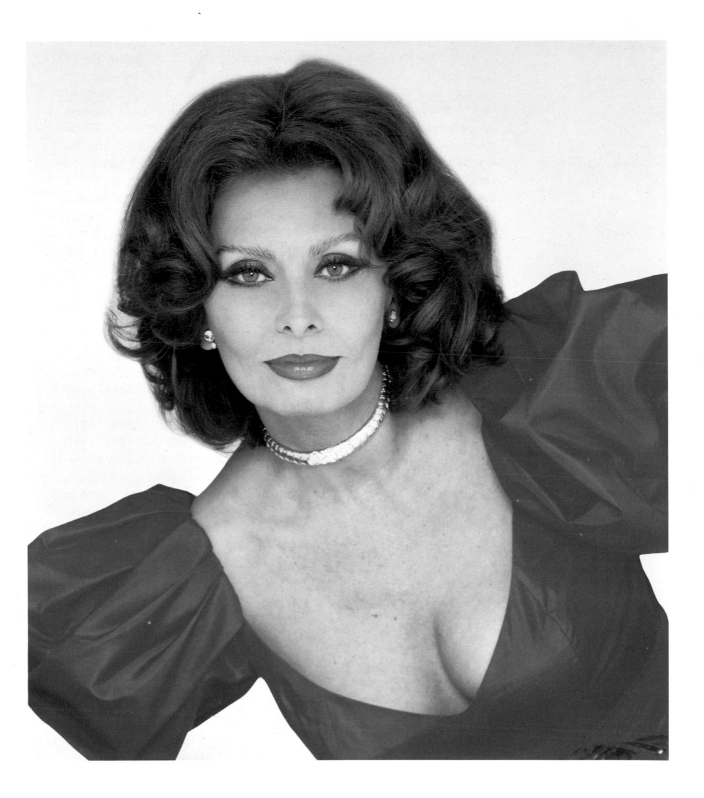

It is a mistake to think that once you are done with school, you need never learn anything new about literature, history, philosophy, music or art. I hope I don't sound like a schoolteacher when I say this. I am merely speaking from my own experience. To my astonishment, the world seems to have grown larger, not smaller, as I have matured. There are so many new and interesting things to do, to see, to learn. I never really used to enjoy museums; now I see why they are such a source of pleasure. I have discovered the theater with a new enthusiasm. I am reading books that I never would have thought of picking up before. Recently I saw a performance of *Romeo and Juliet.* I remembered reading the play at school, and I had seen it performed years ago. But after I left the theater that night, I suddenly realized I had never really known what the play was about. It was not merely a collection of words; it was poetry. And the passion, the emotions of the play had new meaning for me because they were feelings that I too had experienced in my life.

This is the joy of learning new things as an adult: we bring so much more to the process. If you think back to some of the books you read when you were at school, it is hardly surprising that as a child you did not appreciate them. But if you read one today, you will probably be amazed to find what pleasure it brings you.

I think that the women's movement and the atmosphere it has created make this a good time to be a mature woman. Gone forever, I hope, is the idea that once your years of childbearing are past you are of no further use to society. Women are doing things that their mothers would never have dreamed of doing. I consider myself very fortunate to be living in a time when there is always a future for a woman, no matter what her age. But it has to be said that these possibilities exist only for the woman whose mind is growing, who is always prepared to try something new. The woman who spends all her time using makeup to camouflage her wrinkles, dye to disguise her gray hair and exercises to reshape her body will reach a point where she can be nothing but a failure because her goal is an impossible one.

So if you put on a little weight, find that you need glasses, get twinges of pain in your knees, and notice that a few dark-brown spots are showing on your hands, don't despair. There is a fountain of youth: it is your mind, your talents, the creativity you bring to your life and the lives of people you love. When you learn to tap this source, you will truly have defeated age.

INDEX

Page numbers in italic refer to illustrations.